MEDICAL
INTELLIGENCE
UNIT

HIBERNATION INDUCTION TRIGGER FOR ORGAN PRESERVATION

MEDICAL
INTELLIGENCE
UNIT

HIBERNATION INDUCTION TRIGGER FOR ORGAN PRESERVATION

Sufan Chien, M.D.
Peter R. Oeltgen, Ph.D.

University of Kentucky
Lexington

R.G. LANDES COMPANY
AUSTIN

MEDICAL INTELLIGENCE UNIT

HIBERNATION INDUCTION TRIGGER
FOR ORGAN PRESERVATION

R.G. LANDES COMPANY
Austin / Georgetown

CRC Press is the exclusive worldwide distributor of publications of the Medical Intelligence Unit.
CRC Press, 2000 Corporate Blvd., NW, Boca Raton, FL 33431. Phone: 407/994-0555.

Submitted: December 1992
Published: January 1993

Production Manager: Terry Nelson
Copy Editor: Constance Kerkaporta

Please address all inquiries to the Publisher:
R.G. Landes Company
909 Pine Street
Georgetown, TX 78626
or
P.O. Box 4858
Austin, TX 78765
Phone: 512/ 863 7762
FAX: 512/ 863 0081

ISBN 1-879702-34-7
CATALOG # LN0234

Acknowledgements

These studies could not have been completed without the help of our colleagues and helpers. The following people deserve special thanks.

Dr. Byron Young, Professor and Chairman of the Department of Surgery, University of Kentucky Medical Center, is a long-time supporter of this project. Dr. Edward P. Todd and Dr. Robert K. Salley, the former and current chiefs of the Division of Cardiothoracic Surgery, have provided enormous support for all the studies. Without their support, the studies could not have been finished.

Dr. John N. Diana, Professor of Physiology and Biophysics and Director of the Tobacco and Health Research Institute, University of Kentucky, has provided substantial support for the study, not only financially through grant funds but also with his expertise in mammalian physiology. Without his help and support, the study would have proceeded much more slowly.

We also wish to thank the medical technologists at the Lexington VA Medical Center for expertly performing the wide array of chemical and hematological tests required to conduct these studies.

The following people have been involved in our experiments from time to time: Drs. William O'Connor, Michael Sekela, Sheryl Mahony, Todd Marian, Xuejun Shi, David Gross, Richard Maley, Guanghan Wu, Futing Zhang, Zuyi Zhang, Mr. Byron Keith, Miss Laurie Sharp, Ms. Marta Sparks, Ms. Sherrie Lanzo, Mr. Chris Johns, and Mr. Brian Proffitt. The electron microscopy study was provided by Richard Geissler in the Department of Pathology. Each of these individuals was extremely helpful in the enormous task of performing these time-consuming experiments.

Dr. Tsung-Ping Su in NIDA-Addiction Research Center provided technical support for suggesting the use of DADLE in these studies.

We wish to express our special gratitude to Mr. Glenn Proffitt for his technical assistance. Mr. Proffitt not only helped with the surgical preparation, but also devised much of the equipment needed for the preservation studies.

We also wish to express our gratitude to US Surgical for providing the staplers. The various research projects were supported in part by grants from the National Institutes of Health, HL36248, NIH GM43890; the VA Medical Research Fund; the US Army Medical Research and Development Command Contract No. DAMD-17-87-C-7070; and University of Kentucky Research Grants RR05374, 2-03840, 2-04937 and 2-04998.

We would like to acknowledge the encouragement and support provided in editing this text by Ms. Flo Witte, Director of the Publications Office of the Department of Surgery. The illustrations in the Chapter 3 were the fine work of Mr. Richard A. Gersony, Medical Illustrator for the Department of Surgery. We are also grateful to Ms. Sherry Williams of the Publications Office, who checked the references for accuracy.

We wish to express our special appreciation to the publishers of this monograph.

CONTENTS

PREFACE

Successfully transferring tissue and organs from one person to another has been one of the great achievements of modern medicine and surgery. The introduction of cyclosporine represents a further step forward. A challenge still to be overcome, however, is reliably preserving the graft in the interval between procurement and implantation. Successful organ preservation depends upon the balance between metabolic energy requirements, oxygen and nutrient supplies and upon the efficacy of disposing of metabolic waste products. A satisfactory technique for organ preservation must meet several fundamental requirements: controlling the metabolism and energy requirements of the organs, administering necessary nutrients, providing the required oxygen, and removing cellular metabolic waste products. This monograph reports a newly developed autoperfusion multiorgan preparation which seems to meet all these requirements for long-term organ preservation.

Hibernation is a physiologic state characterized by profoundly depressed body temperature, respiration, cardiovascular function and general metabolism. Hibernators avoid freezing and arouse spontaneously to euthermia so that they can control metabolism levels and system function. It is now known that hibernation induction trigger (HIT) obtained from the plasma of winter-hibernating woodchucks, ground squirrels, brown cave bats and black bears can induce hibernation in summer-active hibernators placed in a cold room during a season when these animals do not ordinarily hibernate. Moreover, this "trigger" is not found in the blood of summer-active hibernators. Infusion of the HIT-containing albumin fraction into nonhibernating primates induces profound behavioral and physiologic depression including bradycardia, hypothermia, and hypophagia without significant weight loss, an anesthetized state, and decreased renal function. The aforementioned phenomena could be reversed or retarded by the infusion of the opiate antagonists naloxone and naltrexone. HIT has been shown to cause a significant change in renal function and creatinine clearance. Our studies documented the first reported use of HIT-containing plasma from hibernators and the *delta* opioid, DADLE, which mimics its activity in organ preservation studies. Although the mechanism of their action is still not clear, HIT and DADLE extend tissue survival time substantially in autoperfusion multiorgan preparations and contribute to better preservation of heart function in hypothermic storage.

This monograph provides an overview of the development of the different techniques for organ preservation, the nature of hibernation, the technique of multiple organ block harvesting, and the results of using HIT and DADLE during organ preservation. Due to the complexity of the hibernating state, the nature of hibernation induction trigger is still not known at this point. It is our aim to stimulate more research interests in these areas so that the full potential of these opioid-like molecules can be employed.

Sufan Chien, Associate Professor of Surgery
Peter R. Oeltgen, Associate Professor of Pathology

CHAPTER 1

HIBERNATION—THE NATURAL METABOLIC INHIBITOR

Hibernation in mammals is a unique circannual adaptation allowing certain species, such as the ground squirrel, the woodchuck, the brown cave bat, the European hedgehog and the black bear, to survive extended periods of food deprivation when ambient temperatures may be well below freezing. For example, it has been estimated that by hibernating, ground squirrels conserve up to 88% of the energy that would be required if they remained active during the winter.[1] Moreover, it has been suggested that hibernating animals age at a slower rate then those of the same species which are prevented from undergoing hibernation.[2] Profound metabolic changes accompany hibernation, including respiratory depression, a decline in body temperature, and a cessation of feeding and renal function. These changes may be of great survival benefit to animals that can subsist without food and water for up to five months (up to eight months in the arctic ground squirrel). In most hibernators, except the black bear, body temperatures decline to as low as $4°$ to $6°C$ and even $1°$ or $2°C$ below freezing in the arctic ground squirrel.[3]

Some metabolic changes prior to the onset of hibernation may be due to phosphorylation-mediated enzyme inactivation.[4] During hibernation, stored fat becomes the primary metabolic fuel. Carbohydrate needs are met by gluconeogenesis from amino acids. Urea, the primary nitrogen-containing waste product of protein catabolism, is recycled rather than excreted, thereby negating the need for urination and hence arousal.[5,6] Actively dividing cells, such as those of the intestinal epithelium, become relatively quiescent.[7] However, despite the profound metabolic, biochemical, and cellular changes noted in hibernating animals, relatively little information is available concerning the mechanism(s) that induce and maintain these changes or those involved in reversing them. A major reason for this problem is that most hibernation studies rely on in vivo systems, making experiential manipulation both difficult and expensive.

IDENTIFICATION OF HIBERNATION INDUCTION TRIGGER (HIT) MOLECULE(S)

The suggestion of a trigger substance that actively induces entry into the hibernating state has gained considerable acceptance and has implicated a large number of endogenous substances from a variety of tissues such as brain,[8,9] brown fat,[10] hormones[11] and electrolytes.[12,13] However, it was not until 1969 that

Dawe and Spurrier[14] presented the first direct evidence for the presence of a "trigger" in the blood of hibernating ground squirrels (*Citellus tridecemlineatus*) that can induce natural mammalian hibernation when injected into summer-active animals (a season when these animals do not ordinarily hibernate). Saline-infused control ground squirrels maintained identically to experimental animals in a hibernaculum at $4°$-$6°C$ during the summer failed to hibernate. Similar findings occurred when plasma from hibernating woodchucks (*Marmota monax*) was injected into summer-active ground squirrels or woodchucks without adverse immune response. Studies originating from Bruce's laboratory[15,16] have confirmed the original findings of Dawe and Spurrier and extended them to another true hibernator, the bat. Bruce and co-workers have clearly demonstrated that plasma from two species of hibernating bats (*Myotis licifugus* and *Eptesicus fuscus*) contains a hibernation trigger which can induce hibernation in summer-active ground squirrels. More recently, Bruce et al[17,18] and Ruit et al[19] have shown that a plasma fraction derived from hibernating black bears and female polar bears can act in a similar fashion. The latter finding is significant in that it indicates a common form of HIT in at least four distinct species (woodchuck, ground squirrels, bat and bear). However, the area of specific isolation and chemical characterization of this hibernation induction trigger (HIT) molecule have been until recently virtually unexplored.[20-22] The absence in this area may primarily be attributed to the necessity of using a bioassay requiring induction of hibernation in summer-active ground squirrels or woodchucks (a very restrictive seasonal time frame for testing).

In spite of these major drawbacks, our work over the past years, using three distinct protein resolving techniques (isoelectric focusing,[23] preparative isotachophoresis[24] and affinity chromatography[25]) has given the first real clues about the chemical identify of the HIT molecule. (Figs. 1-3) Our experiments have demonstrated that this molecule is closely bound or associated with albumin and that its physiologic role in hibernators may be dependent upon changing albumin concen-

trations.[26] To date, our studies indicate that the HIT molecule is a small, thermolabile, protease-sensitive, nuclease-insensitive protein possibly in excess of 5,000 M.W.[21] Furthermore, the studies of Spurrier and Dawe,[27] Oeltgen et al[22] and Rotermund and Veltman[28] have greatly expanded our understanding of the physiologic and biochemical effects of the HIT molecule on the circulation and the blood and membrane components of hibernators. Rotermund and Veltman have documented marked changes in membrane lipid compounds of animals in deep hibernation. Especially notable is the higher degree of unsaturation of fatty acids, which would tend to favor greater tissue fluidity at low temperatures. The work of Spurrier and Dawe indicates that erythrocytes of animals in deep hibernation at $4°$-$6°C$ fold over, are more pliable, and easily pass through constricted cap-

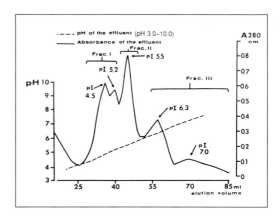

Fig. 1. Separation of hibernating woodchuck plasma by isoelectric focusing in a pH gradient extending from 3.5 -10 using a LKB 8100 Electrofocusing Column. The curve with peaks shows the absorption of the eluted at 280 nm. The steadily increasing curve is a plot of the pH gradient superimposed. Isoelectric point values shown at various peaks were read from the pH gradient curve. The three main plasma fractions were then assayed for biological (HIT) activity in three groups of summer-active ground squirrels, each group comprising 10 animals. Aliquots of fractions I, II and III, at a concentration of 3 mg/ml of 0.9% NaCl, were injected into the saphenous veins of ground squirrels. All animals receiving Fractions II or III failed to hibernate, whereas 8 of 10 ground squirrels receiving Fraction I hibernated within 2-6 days after injection.

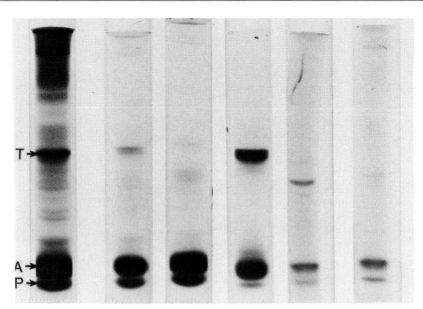

Fig. 2. Polyacrylamide gels of 400 µg aliquots of fractions derived from the plasma of hibernating woodchucks. Each gel is a separation of plasma fractions exhibiting HIT activity (capable of inducing hibernation in summer-active ground squirrels when injected in the saphenous vein at a concentration of 3.0 mg/ml physiologic saline). These fractions, in which albumin predominates, were derived by isoelectric focusing (IEF), isotachophoresis, and affinity chromatography. Gel number 1 represents whole hibernating woodchuck plasma for comparison purposes. Gels 2 and 3 were derived by IEF using pH 3.5-10 and 3.5-6 pH gradients, respectively. Gel 4 represents an albumin fraction derived from a preparative isotachophoresis column and indicates the presence of a distinct transferrin band midway in the gel, whereas Gels 5 and 6 represent affinity chromatography separations from whole hibernating woodchuck plasma and the albumin fraction (Fraction I - Gel number 2) derived by IEF. In every instance, albumin is the predominant protein constituent of fractions that can induce hibernation in summer-active ground squirrels. Abbreviations: A=albumin, P=pre albumin, T=transferrin.

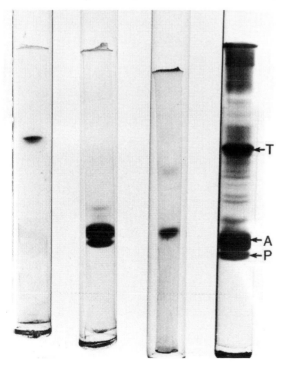

Fig. 3. (Left) Even the relatively homogeneous HIT-containing fractions derived from the affinity chromatography technique (Gels 5 & 6, Fig. 2) and from the preparative isotachophoresis technique (Gel 4, Fig. 2) contained transferrin. Therefore, we applied the albumin fraction from the affinity columns to a preparative gel electrophoretic column for further purification. Analytical polyacrylamide gel electrophoresis of fractions 1, 2 and 3 derived by preparative gel electrophoresis on the LKB Uniphor (LKB Instruments, Stockholm, Sweden) are compared to whole woodchuck plasma. Bioassay results indicated that five of five summer-active ground squirrels hibernated when injected with 3 mg/ml of fraction 1, whereas three of five hibernated when injected with Fraction 2 and zero of five hibernated when injected with Fraction 3, which contained only transferrin and thus effectively ruled out this globulin as the plasma-binding protein for the HIT molecule.

illary beds providing tissues with oxygen. This is quite unlike the process seen in nonhibernators exposed to similar temperatures. In these animals erythrocytes stack up in rouleau formation and cannot negotiate constricted capillary beds. Our experiments[22] using an isoelectric focusing technique to characterize the hemoglobin of ground squirrels in various activity states indicate significant qualitative changes in the hemoglobin molecules formed during natural and HIT-induced summer hibernation. Possibly, the erythropoietic tissues respond to naturally produced or injected HIT by synthesizing hemoglobin molecules that can more readily dissociate oxygen to hypothermic tissues. The aforementioned changes would most likely be of great survival benefit for these animals that can subsist without food and water for up to five months while body temperatures decline to 4°-6°C, heart rates to 1 or 2 beats per minute and respirations to one or two per minute, and urine production to zero during natural-winter or summer-induced hibernation.

The Effect of the Hibernation Induction Trigger (HIT) Molecule on Nonhibernating Recipients

Although HIT has previously been shown to exert a highly specific effect in an environmentally adapted hibernating species, our experiments employing a primate model (*Macaca mulatta*) indicate that infusing the HIT molecule initiates a sequence of dramatic physiologic and behavioral effects in a species that is not able to undergo hibernation.

These studies indicate that intracerebroventricular (ICV) infusion of the isolated HIT-containing albumin fraction from hibernating woodchucks into conscious chaired primates can produce opiate-like behavioral modifications[29] and initiate profound behavioral and physiologic depression marked by hypothermia, bradycardia and long-term hypophagia.[30-32] Intravenous infusions of albumin fractions derived from winter-hibernating but not summer-active woodchucks initiate quite comparable responses and dramatically alter primate renal function as evidenced by marked decreases in creatinine clearance and urine flow.[33]

In the primate experiments, adult male (n=3) and female (n=3) rhesus monkeys weighing 6-8 and 3.5-5.5 kg, respectively, were adapted to primate restraining chairs located in an experimental room with an ambient temperature of 22°-24°C and an illumination cycle of 15 h light and 9 h dark. The monkeys were maintained on ad lib. supply of water and were trained to press a lever activating a mouth feeder that delivered specially formulated 0.3 g banana pellets (P. J. Noyes Co., Precision Food Pellets, Lancaster, NH).

The neurosurgical procedures for cannula and thermistor implantation in the primates were as follows:

Male animals were sedated with ketamine hydrochloride (15 mg/kg) and were anesthetized with gaseous halothane prior to surgical manipulation. The ovariectomized female monkeys were anesthetized by sodium pentobarbital (25-30 mg/kg) injected into the saphenous vein. Cardiac electrodes for monitoring heart rate and blood pressure were placed as previously described.[34] In the male rhesus monkeys, continuous core measurements were available after a 5 mm craniotomy hole was aseptically drilled in the parietal bone and a YSI 42 thermistor probe (Yellow Springs Instrument Co.) was inserted 1 cm subdurally. The thermistor was cemented with cranioplast and anchored to stainless steel screws drilled into the skull. In the earlier female monkey experiments, a thermistor was inserted into the colon of each monkey to a depth of 10 cm so that body temperature could be monitored continuously prior to each experiment. ECG, heart rate, core temperature and blood pressure were monitored on a Beckman R611 polygraph. The head of the anesthetized animal was placed in a stereotaxic instrument, and an 18-gauge stainless steel cannula[35] affixed to a Collison base was screwed into the skull bilaterally according to rigid aseptic procedures described previously.[36]

Following an incision in the midline, two holes were drilled equidistantly 6-7 mm from the mid-sagittal suture at an AP coordinate of 12-14 mm anterior to stereotaxic 0. After each hole was threaded by a tap, the cannula was screwed into the skull so that the tip rested 10-12 mm below the surface of the dura. A 20-gauge inner cannula connected to a 50-cm length of PE-60 tubing was inserted through the diaphragm of a Collison cap. Cannula placement, patency determination, and the preparation of an artificial 5-ion cerebrospinal fluid (CSF) control infusion were carried out according to the rigid aseptic procedures described by Myers[35] and Myers et al.[36] The animals were permitted 10 days to two weeks to recover from the surgical procedures. In experiments using male rhesus monkeys, overt primate behavioral patterns before and after ICV and IV injection of control or HIT-containing albumin fractions were monitored by a television camera and recorded on videotape. The homogenity of 400 μg aliquots of all these fractions was determined by analytical polyacrylamide gel electrophoresis using the standard methodology of Davis.[37] Gels were stained with Coomassie Blue as previously described.[38]

The affinity chromatographic technique, employing Affi-Gel Blue as the chromatography matrix, was used to obtain nearly homogeneous HIT-containing albumin fractions for ICV and IV infusions in primates and has been detailed previously.[25] Prior to ICV infusion, these fractions were dissolved in an artificial cerebrospinal fluid (CSF) containing Na^+ (127.6 mM), K^+ (2.5 mM), Ca^{++} (1.26 mM), Mg^{++} (0.93 mM), and Cl_2 (134.58 mM)[35]. The fractions were rendered sterile by passing them through a 0.21 μ Amicon Sterilet (Amicon, Danvers, MA).

For earlier female rhesus studies, control infusions of either 5-ion CSF or bovine serum albumin (BSA) were used, the latter in the same mg/μl concentrations as fractions derived from hibernating or summer-active woodchuck plasma. In addition, 100 mg of norepinephrine (NE) HCl was infused ICV to a concentration of 25 μg/100 μl to serve as a functional hypothermic check of ventricular patency. In the later experiments using male rhesus monkeys, the 5-ion CSF and monkey serum albumin (MSA) were used for control infusions prior to HIT administration.

As depicted for a representative male rhesus monkey in Figure 4, infusing 8.0 ml of the HIT-containing albumin fraction in 400 μl of 5-ion CSF into the lateral ventricle exerted a profound effect on the behavioral patterns and physiologic parameters of chaired, conscious monkeys. The sequential behavioral responses, which usually ensued within 10-15 min following infusions, were retching, yawning, mouth gaping and extreme lethargy, followed by eye closure, head slumping and appearance of an anesthetized state for 3-5 hours. Physiologic responses included a marked hypothermia of varying intensity, onset and duration (1.5° to 3°C from baseline, mean fall in brain temperature equals 2.6°C); a coinciding bradycardia extending up to 8 hours postinfusion (average maximal decrease 43%-50% from baseline, mean decrease equals 45.6%); and a clear-cut hypophagic period lasting up to 5-7 days with no food intake at all during the first 12-18 hours. We also noted that there was virtually no weight loss during the hypophagic period in the three male animals studied. Although fluid intake and urine production were not monitored, we noted that the bedding of the animals was virtually urine free during the first few days following the HIT infusion. None of the aforementioned behavioral or physiologic responses was evident when 400 μl of 5-ion artificial CSF vehicle or 8 mg of monkey serum albumin (MSA) were infused.

The earlier experiments with female rhesus monkeys, in which we infused 4.0 mg of HIT-albumin from summer-active woodchucks (SAWA) and bovine serum albumin (BSA) along with 5-ion CSF, resulted in essentially similar but less dramatic behavioral and physiologic depression in these animals. A representative decline in body temperature following the 4-mg dose of HIT is shown in Figure 5. As illustrated in the figure, the hypothermic episode began almost immediately and continued for nearly four hours. Then the temperature returned rapidly to baseline level. (Fig. 5 top) By comparison, an injection of 100 μg NE into the same ventricular cannula caused the typical catecholaminergic hypothermia characterized by a very rapid fall and a short-lived nadir. Control infusions of 5-ion CSF and 4 mg of SAWA and BSA caused no hypothermia, bradycardia, or behavioral modifications. In another female monkey a deep hypothermia began

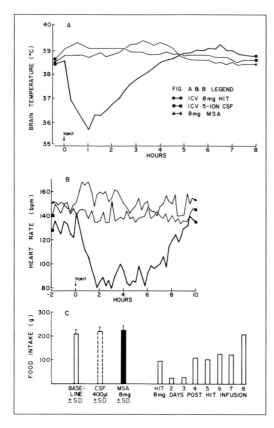

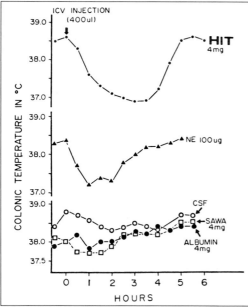

Fig. 5. Colonic temperature of a representative female rhesus monkey following ICV injection in each experiment, in a volume of 400 µl of 4 mg HIT (top); 100 µg NE (middle); or 5-ion CSF, 4 mg of SAWA or 4 mg BSA (bottom). Abscissa is time in hours.

about 24 hours after 4 mg in 400 µl of HIT was injected into the primate's ventricle. A hypothermia of 1.5°-2°C persisted for about 4 days, during which time heart rate dropped intermittently from a basal level of 150-160 beats per min to 90-100 beats per min. Although the respiratory rate was essentially unaffected, reflexes were substantially depressed, and the animal became lethargic and aphagic.

An overall analysis revealed that the HIT evoked a mean fall in colonic temperature of 1.02°C (n=3), NE a decline of 1.36°C (n=3), and SAWA a mean increase in temperature of 0.2°C (n=3).

The patterns of food intake and the total number of banana pellets consumed over 24

Fig. 4. (Top, left) Physiological responses after HIT (●—●), MSA (▲—▲) and 5-ion CSF (■—■) infusion in the conscious monkey. The physiologic responses of an individual primate rather than those for all three animals are presented because the onset, extent and duration of hypothermia, bradycardia and hypophagia varied from animal to animal, thereby obscuring somewhat the phenomena in a composite analysis.
(A) Brain temperature of a representative male rhesus monkey following ICV injection of 8 mg HIT in 400 µl artificial CSF, 400 µl of CSF 5-ion vehicle, and 8 mg MSA in 400 µl CSF. The MSA was isolated identically to the HIT albumin fraction using an affinity chromatography column with AFFI-GEL Blue as the chromatography matrix. All preparations were infused over a two-minute period. Serum immunoglobulin and levels of CSF-protein and glucose were determined before and at the end of each agreement. No significant changes in these parameters were noted following HIT or MSA injections.
(B) Heart rate (15-min computer averages) of a representative monkey. An interval of 48 hours or longer was maintained between each ICV injection in a volume of 400 µl CSF, 8 mg MSA or 8 mg HIT. Abscissa is time in hours.
(C) Intake of banana pellets of a representative monkey whose baseline intake over five days was 208 g (left). At an interval of 48 hours or longer, 400 µl CSF vehicle (2nd from left), 8 mg MSA (3rd from left), and 8 mg HIT (4th from left) were infused into the lateral brain ventricle over a two-minute period in 400 µl of 5-ion CSF. The long-term hypophagic response lasting seven days post-HIT infusion is also noted on the abscissa.

hours by the female monkeys varied considerably from monkey to monkey, but in each case a clear-cut hypophagic period ensued after HIT infusions. A moderate hypophagia compared to controls was noted after infusing 4 mg SAWA in one animal, but this response was absent in the other two. The latter finding may indicate that low residual levels of HIT activity are present in hibernating animals year-round. Figure 6 illustrates the 24-hour feeding patterns and hypophagic response for one female monkey.

The aforementioned primate behavioral modifications and hypophagia were reminiscent of an opioid-like state.[39] Moreover, the first indication that the HIT molecule may exert its effect through an opioid mechanism(s) appeared in evidence presented by Beckman et al.[40] These authors observed that, when morphine sulfate tablets that had been inserted subcapsularly in summer-active and winter-hibernating ground squirrels were removed after six weeks, only the summer-active animals exhibited the typical "abstinence syndrome." It was possible that the resistance of hibernating ground squirrels but not active animals to the physical dependence on morphine may have been due to the blocking of brain opioid receptor sites by endogenous opioid peptides such as the HIT molecule. It is quite conceivable that the HIT molecule might represent a naturally occurring form of opioid agonist or antagonist.

Based on our primate experimental observations and Beckman's study, we decided to use either the short-acting opiate antagonist naloxone (Endo Laboratories) IV following ICV infusion of HIT or the long-acting opiate antagonist naltrexone (Endo Laboratories) ICV prior to ICV HIT infusions.

Intravenous infusion of naloxone (30 μg/kg) one hour after infusion of 8 mg of HIT had a remarkable effect in all three male monkeys in that the animals became alert and oriented within minutes. Naloxone completely abolished the long-term hypophagic response; in some cases animals began immediate feeding. Moreover, the opiate antagonist attenuated the hypothermic response and the extent and duration of bradycardia. (Fig. 7) Infusion of 200 μg in 200 μl of 5-ion CSF of the long-

acting opiate antagonist naltrexone one hour prior to HIT infusion delayed the onset of the hypothermic response by over an hour and also limited its extent. Unlike naloxone, naltrexone also abolished the bradycardia. Also, the animals experienced only brief episodes of lethargy and eye closure and no long-term hypophagia. Intravenous control injections of naloxone or ICV infusions of naltrexone resulted in no behavioral modifications or significant physiologic alterations.

Initial experiments in which chaired female monkeys (n=3) were infused IV with either 10 mg of HIT or control infusions of 10 mg SAWA or BSA in 10 ml of physiologic

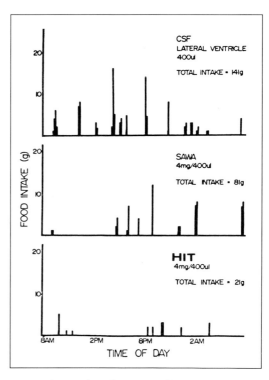

Fig. 6. The intake of banana pellets by a representative female rhesus monkey over individual one-day periods following ICV injection in a volume of 400 μl of: 5-ion artificial CSF (top); 4 mg of SAWA (middle); or 4 mg of HIT (bottom). The total food consumed over 24 hours is noted in each case; a slight hypophagic response was noted even after ICV injection of 4 mg SAWA (middle). Food intake declined to 81 g compared to 141 g for CSF (top), but this was not nearly as marked a hypophagia as occurred when 4 mg HIT were infused ICV (bottom), dropping food intake to 21 g.

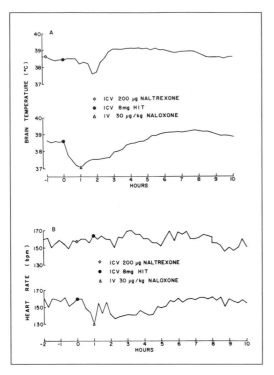

Fig. 7. The effects of the opiate antagonists naloxone (-△-) and naltrexone (-◇-) on the core temperature and heart rate of the conscious monkey either one hour before or after injection of HIT (-●-).

(A) Top curve indicates the one-hour delay and moderation of the hypothermic response caused by injecting 200 µg of the long acting opiate antagonist naltrexone one hour prior to injection of 8 mg HIT. Bottom curve depicts the moderating influence on hypothermic response one hour after IV injection of naloxone (30 µg/kg).

(B) Top curve indicates the abolition of bradycardia by ICV injection of naltrexone one hour prior to HIT injection. Bottom curve indicates the attenuation of bradycardia after injection of naloxone (30 µg/kg) one hour following injection of 8 mg HIT.

Fig. 8. (Right) Intake of food of a representative female rhesus monkey over individual one-day periods. A hypophagic response occurred following intravenous infusion of 10 mg of HIT in 1 ml of physiologic saline into the saphenous vein (bottom). Food intake dropped to 154 g/d as compared to 10 mg BSA (top) 232 g/d and SAWA (middle) 218 g/d, both of which had virtually no effect on food intake.

saline indicated that the HIT molecule can exert a dramatic hypophagic response by this route of administration, as shown for a representative animal in Figure 8. Based on these observations, we gave 50 mg doses of the HIT fraction in 2.5 ml of physiologic saline to two caged male monkeys. In both animals the response was immediate and included an apparent peripheral ischemia and the aforementioned ICV behavioral responses. However, these unchaired animals could not maintain equilibrium, toppled, and lay on their bellies or sides with their eyes closed. They were virtually areflexive (for three hours in one animal and five hours in the second). Figure 9 indicates that a long-term hypophagic response lasted approximately three weeks in each animal before feeding returned to baseline levels. Remarkably, neither animal lost more than 200 grams of weight, and urine output was markedly reduced because bedding needed infrequent changes. In other studies[21] using three male rhesus monkeys, we noticed an almost 40% decrease in 24 hr creatinine clearance, marked reductions in urine flow, and a tendency toward decreased creatinine production as compared to baseline levels following IV infusions of 50 mg of HIT

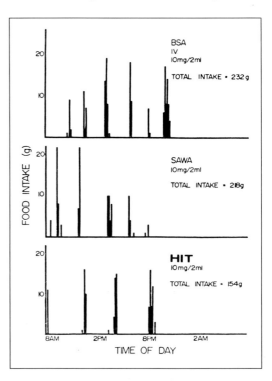

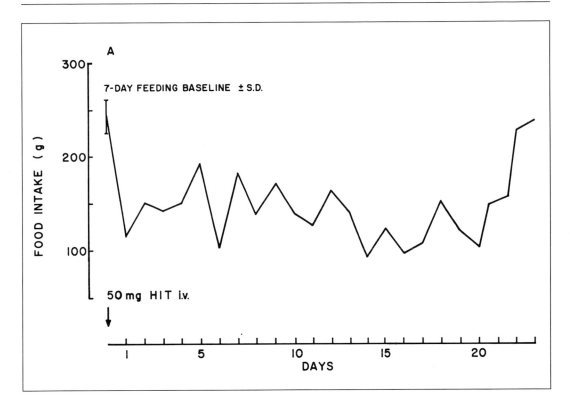

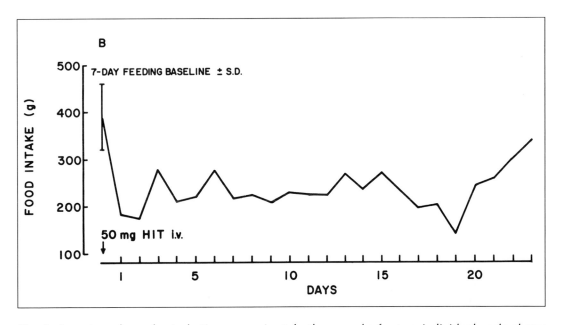

Fig. 9. Long-term hypophagia lasting approximately three weeks for two individual male rhesus monkeys (A & B) following intravenous injection into the saphenous vein of 50 mg of HIT-containing albumin fraction derived from the affinity chromatography column. The IV infusion resulted in an immediate behavioral and physiologic depression similar to that noted for ICV HIT infusions. The seven-day feeding baseline for monkey A was 243 ± 16 g, while that for monkey B was 386 ± 54 g. The mean hypophagic response in monkey A over a 21-day time span was 135 ± 27 g (46% feeding decline compared to 7-day feeding baseline). Saline injections had no effect on feeding in either monkey.

Table 1. Renal function parameters (Mean ± SD)

	Creatinine Clearance	Urine Flow Rate	Creatinine Production
Control	32.5 ± 4.2	0.183 ± 0.072	0.287 ± 0.055
HIT	19.7 ± 1.8*	0.061 ± 0.008	0.230 ± 0.023
SAWA	30.3 ± 1.7	0.156 ± 0.046	0.274 ± 0.057

*$p < 0.05$; HIT vs. SAWA

fractions derived from the affinity chromatography column. (Table 1) Comparably isolated summer-active albumin fractions did not significantly alter primate renal function when compared to baseline levels.

Because of the significant reductions in creatinine clearance (a most sensitive and reliable indicator of kidney function and catabolic protein breakdown process in the body) and the reduced urine flow and creatinine production following HIT infusion, it seems quite reasonable to assume that, in addition to the hypothermia, aphagia, and opioid-like behavioral depression induced by HIT, the albumin fraction (and its associated HIT) present endogenously in the woodchuck during winter hibernation exerts a direct action on the kidney of the primate, possibly on the mechanisms underlying glomerular filtration and the tubular reabsorption process. Further evidence substantiating this theory is that in hibernating bears metabolic wastes do not accumulate because of reincorporation of labeled amino acids into tissue protein.[6] Because such dramatic decreases in basal metabolic activity occur in the hibernator, one would anticipate that a mechanism(s) exists to conserve lean body mass in the animal in hibernation. Thus, the necessity for renal function (glomerular filtration and urine production) is obviated. Because the HIT molecule is more purified, such depressions in the renal function of nonhibernators could be expected to be even more profound and could have long-term organ-sparing consequences.

We have also infused 10 mg of HIT in 400 µl of saline into the lateral ventricles of three female beagle dogs weighing 8-10 kg in an effort to document the suspected but unverifiable analgesia we observed in primates that had received the HIT preparation. In this yet unpublished experiment, we used the standardized skin twitch reflex analgesic testing system of Hardy et al[41] as modified by Martin et al[42,43] and Wettstein et al.[44] These dogs exhibited a long-term analgesic response beginning 30-45 minutes after HIT infusion and lasting 4-6 hours. Other responses noted were opiate-like retching at 15-20 minutes after infusion, rhinorrhea, markedly decreased respirations (10-12 per minute versus 18-30 normal), and long-term feeding inhibition. None of the aforementioned responses were observed with summer-active woodchuck albumin fractions.

CHARACTERIZATION OF HIT OPIOID-LIKE EFFECTS IN NONHIBERNATING RECIPIENTS

Because most of the aforementioned behavioral and physiologic depressions noted in primates can be blocked or retarded by IV or ICV infusion of the opiate antagonists naloxone and naltrexone, we now have reason to suspect that the HIT molecule is either opiate in nature or a neuropeptide hormone that initiates its action through opioid receptor(s).[30] We have also shown that the opioid antagonist naloxone,[17] the *kappa* agonist U69593[45] and the *mu* agonists morphine and morphiceptin, as well as the naturally occurring *kappa* brain opioid agonist dynorphin, can all block hibernation induced by HIT when infused via mini-osmotic pumps implanted subscapularly in summer-active ground squirrels.[46,47] Only the *delta* opioid D-Ala^2-D-Leu^5-Enkephalin (DADLE) induced hibernation in summer-active ground squirrels in a fashion similar to that observed in animals injected with HIT and saline in infusion pumps.[46,47] The inhibitory action on summer-induced hibernation by the opioid antagonist naloxone is shown in Figure 10, whereas that of the highly specific *kappa* agonist U-69593 is depicted in Figure 11 and

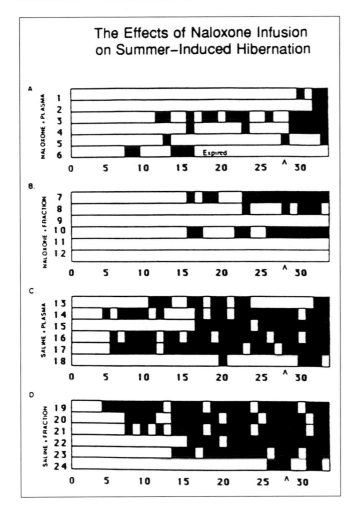

The Effects of Naloxone Infusion on Summer–Induced Hibernation

Fig. 10. Patterns of summer hibernation in 13 lined ground squirrels following subscapular osmotic minipump placement containing naloxone A & B or saline C & D. Group A received whole hibernating black bear plasma whereas Group B received HIT-containing albumin fraction from black bears. Groups C & D received whole back bear plasma and the HII-containing albumin fraction, respectively.

those of the naturally occurring brain *kappa* opioid dynorphin A and the *mu* agonists morphine and morphiceptin are depicted in Figures 12 and 13. The hibernation induction capacity of the *delta* opioid DADLE is depicted in Figures 14 and 15.

DEVELOPMENT OF A RAPID IN VITRO BIOASSAY TO FACILITATE PURIFICATION OF THE HIT MOLECULE AND RELATED FACTORS

We have recently developed a rapid in vitro assay system used for both purifying and characterizing HIT-like molecules present in the plasma of hibernating woodchucks. This system, which replaces the seasonally restrictive ground squirrel bioassay, measures inhibition of DNA and protein synthesis (metabolic inhibition at the cellular level) and unusual changes in calcium levels in cul-

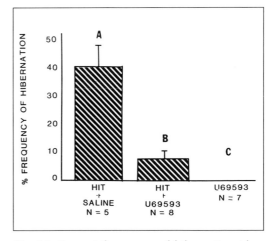

Fig. 11. Percent frequency of hibernation (days spent in hibernation versus total observation days) induced by HIT, HIT combined with U69593 and U69593 alone in summer-active ground squirrels. Opioids were delivered via osmotic minipumps.

tured cells exposed to these molecules. Three cell lines are used for this in vitro bioassay system: 1) TRMP—a dog kidney epithelial cell line;[48] 2) CREF—a rat embryo fibroblast cell line;[49] and 3) SB3—a human kidney tumor (Wilm's) cell line.

Although we have previously reported that an albumin fraction from hibernating woodchuck plasma could induce hibernation in summer-active ground squirrels,[20] we decided to develop the in vitro assay system with unfractionated plasma. This approach allowed us to define a number of the activities of this plasma. Some of these activities may be due to molecules capable of lowering or stimulating cellular metabolism but not capable of inducing hibernation in summer-active animals. Therefore, this new approach may allow us to identify and ultimately purify relevant molecules that would not have been detected with the in vivo bioassay.

To monitor the inhibition of DNA synthesis, we used two separate assays. In the first, the cells were serum starved for 24 hours and then restimulated with 5% fetal bovine serum (FBS) in the presence of various concentrations of plasma obtained from winter-hibernating or summer-active woodchucks.

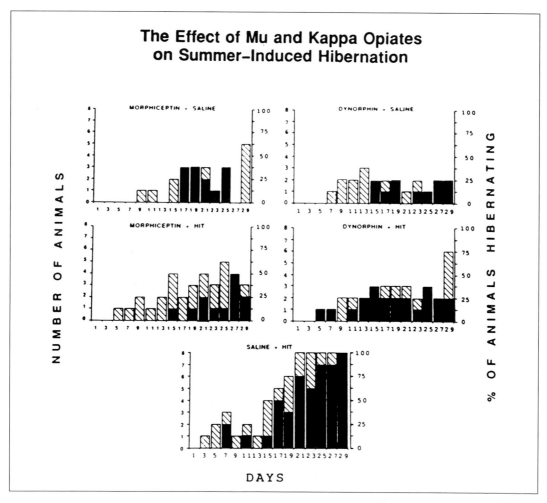

Fig. 12A: Effects on summer-active ground squirrels of morphiceptin in the osmotic pumps and saline injection.
Fig. 12B: Effects of morphiceptin in osmotic pumps and HIT injection.
Fig. 12C: Effects of dynorphin in the osmotic pumps and saline injection.
Fig. 12D: Effects of dynorphin in the osmotic pumps and HIT injection.
For comparison purposes, Fig. 12E depicts the effects of saline in the osmotic pumps and HIT injection.

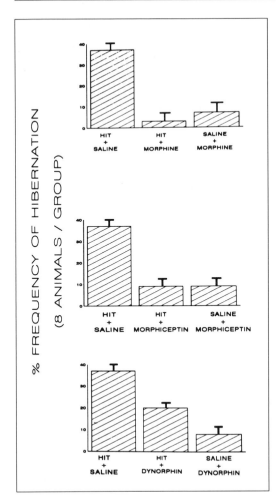

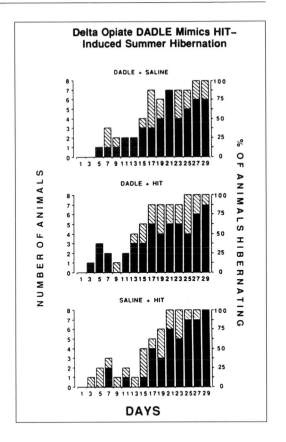

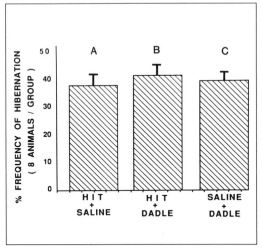

Fig. 13. (Top left) Percent frequency of hibernation (days spent in hibernation versus total observation days) induced by HIT, HIT combined with opioids, and the opioids alone. The % frequency of hibernation of the morphine + saline group was 7.5% ± 2.4%. The morphine + HIT group had a % frequency of hibernation of 0.83% ± 0.83%. The % frequency of hibernation for both the morphine + saline group and the morphiceptin + HIT group was 10.0% ± 2.7%. The dynorphin A + saline group had a % frequency of hibernation of 16.7% ± 3.4%. The % frequency of hibernation in the control group (HIT + saline) was 36.7% ± 4.4%. All groups had a probability less than 0.0001.

Fig. 14. (Top right) Effects of DADLE and DADLE in combination with HIT injection on summer-active ground squirrels. DADLE was delivered through osmotic mini pumps at a rate of 1.50 mg/kg/day. See legend in Fig. 13 for details of the explanation.

Fig. 15. The percent frequency of hibernation induced by HIT plus saline (A), HIT plus DADLE (B), and saline plus DADLE (C) in summer-active ground squirrels. The % frequency of hibernation induced by DADLE+saline was 37.5% ± 4.4%; whereas the DADLE+HIT group had a slightly higher % frequency of 41.7% ± 4.5%.

Figure 16 depicts results with the TRMP cells and Figure 17 with the CREF cells, demonstrating the complete to partial inhibition of the FBS-stimulated DNA synthesis observed with the winter plasma (WWP). For the CREF cells, even at a concentration as low as 0.5% winter-hibernating plasma, significant inhibition of FBS-stimulated DNA synthesis was observed. For both cell lines, equivalent concentrations of the summer-active plasma (WSP) enhanced the FBS stimulation of DNA synthesis. For the second assay, continuously growing cells were exposed to various concentrations of winter plasma, and DNA synthesis was measured every hour for six hours. Figure 18 demonstrates that with the CREF cells DNA synthesis slowed and eventually halted in these cells in a concen-

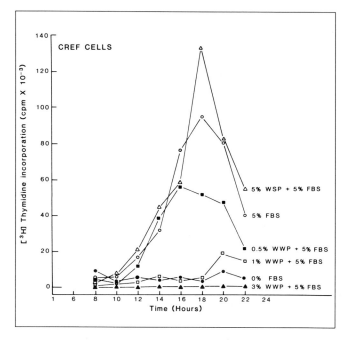

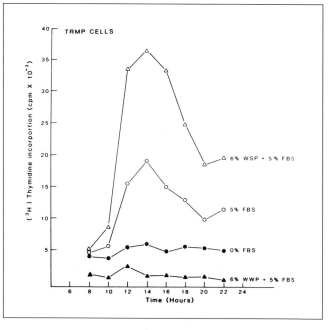

Fig. 16. Complete to partial inhibition of FBS-stimulated DNA synthesis in CREF cells exposed to WWP. Serum-starved CREF cells stimulated by 5% FBS also showed increased incorporation of ³H-thymidine beginning at 10-12 h with a peak at 16-18 h. When supplemented with winter plasma at 5% or 3% (as shown), the ³H-thymidine incorporation was totally inhibited. Partial inhibition was observed at concentrations as low as 0.5% of winter plasma. Summer plasma at 5% with 5% FBS enhanced ³H-thymidine uptake above that observed for 5% FBS alone. This experiment demonstrated that the CREF cells were extremely sensitive to inhibition by winter woodchuck plasma.

Fig. 17. Complete to partial inhibition of FBS-stimulated DNA synthesis in TRMP cells exposed to winter woodchuck plasma (WWP). Plasma from winter-hibernating woodchucks inhibited fetal bovine serum (FBS) stimulation of DNA synthesis in serum-starved TRMP cells. Serum-starved TRMP cells stimulated with 5% FBS show increased incorporation of ³H-thymidine beginning at 10-12 h with a maximum of 16-18 h. When supplemented with 6% winter plasma (as shown), the incorporation of ³H-thymidine was inhibited, falling to a level below that seen for cells maintained in 0% FBS. However, summer plasma at the same concentration (6%) enhanced incorporation of ³H-thymidine above that seen for 5% FBS alone. Similar results were obtained for winter and summer plasma at 7.5% and 5%, demonstrating the presence of an inhibitory factor in the winter woodchuck plasma.

tration-dependent manner. Although not shown in this figure, the summer-active plasma did not inhibit DNA synthesis. To monitor inhibition of protein synthesis, we also used continuously growing cells. The winter plasma was found to inhibit protein synthesis, but equivalent amounts of summer plasma did not. Figure 19 demonstrates these results for the TRMP cells.

The above results with serum-starved cells stimulated with FBS and summer plasma suggested that the summer plasma may also play a role in the stimulation of DNA synthesis. (Figs. 16 and 17) To test this hypothesis, we stimulated serum-starved TRMP cells with concentrations of summer plasma ranging from 0.5%-5% in the absence of FBS and found significant stimulation (not shown).

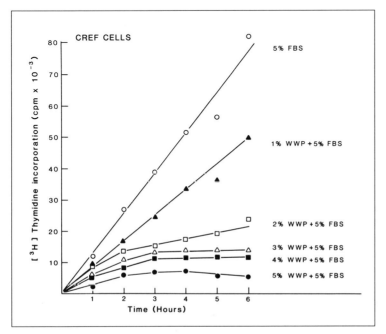

Fig. 18. DNA synthesis measured every 6 hours in continuously growing CREF cells exposed to various concentrations of WWP. Plasma from winter-hibernating woodchucks inhibits DNA synthesis in continuously growing CREF cells. CREF cells growing in DMEM supplemented with 5% FBS were treated with varying concentrations of winter plasma. Significant inhibition of ^{3}H-thymidine incorporation was observed. The level of inhibition was directly proportional to the concentration of winter plasma added, and significant inhibition was observed at concentrations as low as 1%.

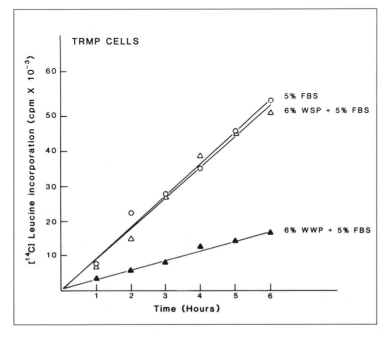

Fig. 19. Inhibition of protein synthesis in TRMP cells following addition of 6% WWP to culture media and absence of protein synthesis inhibition following addition of 6% WSP. Plasma from winter-hibernating woodchucks inhibits protein synthesis in continuously growing TRMP cells. TRMP cells growing in DMEM supplemented with 5% FBS were treated with 6% each of summer and winter woodchuck plasma in the presence of ^{14}C-leucine. Decreased incorporation of ^{14}C-leucine was observed with the 6% winter plasma relative to that seen with both 6% summer plasma plus 5% FBS or with 5% FBS alone.

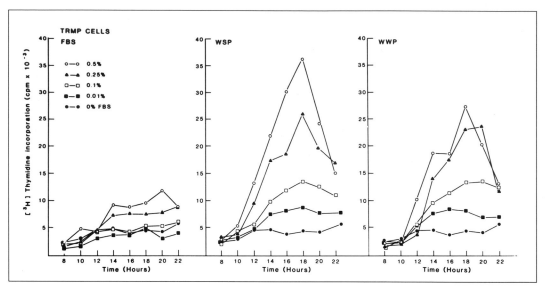

Fig. 20. Stimulation of DNA syntheses in TRMP cells exposed to WSP and WWP at concentrations as low as 0.01%. Low concentrations of plasma from both winter-hibernating and summer-active woodchucks stimulated DNA synthesis in serum-starved TRMP cells. Serum-starved TRMP cells treated with summer or winter woodchuck plasma at concentrations ranging from 0.5%-0.01% were stimulated to incorporate ^{3}H-thymidine. FBS at this low concentration demonstrated only marginal stimulation of ^{3}H-thymidine. This would indicate the presence of a mitogen in both summer and winter woodchuck plasma. However, the mitogen in the winter plasma was revealed upon dilution.

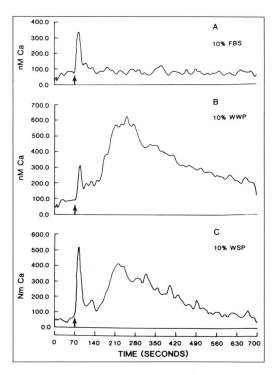

Fig. 21. Calcium response of serum-starved TRMP cells exposed to 10% FBS (Fig. 21A), to 10% winter hibernating woodchuck plasma and (Fig. 21B), and to 10% WSP (Fig. 21C).

This demonstrated that the woodchuck summer-active plasma contained potent mitogenic activity. The detection of such activity in the summer plasma was quite surprising, because plasma from most species, relative to serum, is mitogen poor.[50] Identical experiments with winter-hibernating plasma demonstrated that, at concentrations as low as 2%, DNA synthesis did not occur in the TRMP cells. However, when the plasma concentration was dropped to 0.5%, the winter plasma displayed significant mitogenic activity. Figure 20 demonstrates that both summer-active and winter-hibernating plasma could stimulate detectable amounts of DNA synthesis in the TRMP cells at concentrations as low as 0.01%, whereas FBS could not stimulate DNA synthesis at concentrations below 0.25%.

When serum-starved cells are restimulated with FBS, the first measurable response is a transient intracellular release of stored calcium.[51] This response occurs within seconds, followed by a biphasic pump-down of the free intracellular calcium. Figure 21A demonstrates the calcium response of serum-starved TRMP cells to 10% FBS, Figure 21B to 10% winter-hibernating plasma, and Figure 21C to 10% summer-active plasma. Several significant observations were noted in our experiments. The winter plasma stimulated an initial intracellular calcium release similar to that observed for the FBS, but this was followed by a second, prolonged peak representing the accumulation of intracellular calcium. We have now tested a number of winter-hibernating plasmas, and this second calcium peak has always been observed. The summer plasma stimulated a greater intracellular calcium release than either FBS or winter plasma and was also followed by a second calcium peak. However, this second peak was significantly lower than that observed for the winter plasma.

With the establishment of this in vitro system, we have begun work to determine whether this system will function as a bioassay for purifying both the inhibitory (HIT-active) and mitogenic activities present in the woodchuck plasmas. In these experiments, both sum-mer-active and winter-hibernating plasmas are passed over an Affi-Gel Blue affinity column, and three fractions are collected: the pass-through, proteins removed from the column with 0.2M sodium phosphate, and proteins eluted with 1.4 M NaCl. The last fraction is dialyzed after collection. Table 2 demonstrates that the bulk of the inhibitory activity from the winter-hibernating plasma is eluted with high salt. This fraction is enriched for albumin.[20] Table 3 demonstrates that the bulk of the mitogenic activity from both the summer-active and winter-hibernating plasma is also eluted in this peak, although significant amounts are also found in the other fractions when the TRMP cells are used as a target. We have not yet tested these fractions for inhibition of protein synthesis or their effect on calcium release. Nonetheless, it should be clear that our in vitro assay system will prove useful for purifying these biologically active molecules and characterizing their effect at the cellular levels.

Table 2. Inhibition of DNA synthesis by Affigel-blue column fractions[a]
% Inhibition[b]

Frac.[a]	TRMP	Cells	CREf	Cells	SB3	Cells
wpf[c]	spf[d]	wpf	spf	wpf	spf	
0	100	0	100	7	100	0
1	4	0	39	27	95	16
2	48	18	0	52	0	0
3	100	30	100	35	100	5

a: Serum-starved cells were stimulated with 5% FBS in the presence of 7.5% plasma or concentrated fractions from the Affigel-Blue column.
b: DNA synthesis was measured by determining 3H-thymidine incorporation during the interval of 12-18 hrs after FBS stimulation. The % inhibition was determined by comparing the amount of thymidine incorporation in the presence of the different column fractions with the amount observed with 5% FBS alone.
c: wpf = protein fractions obtained from the winter-hibernating plasma.
d: spf = protein fractions obtained from the summer-active plasma.
e: The tested fractions are as follows: 0 = unfractionated plasma, 1 = protein that passed through the column, 2 = protein that was weakly bound to the column and removed with the 0.02M phosphate buffer, 3 = protein eluted with 1.4M NaCl (albumin fraction).

Table 3. Stimulation of DNA synthesis by Affigel-blue column fractions[a]
% Stimulation[b]

Frac.[a]	TRMP	Cells	CREF	Cells
	wpfc	spf[d]	wpf	spf
0	133	108	127	112
1	105	30	17	1
2	78	0	17	1
3	94	83	95	75

a: Serum-starved cells were stimulated with 0.5% plasma or concentrated plasma protein fractions
b: DNA synthesis was measured by determining 3H-thymidine incorporation at 12-18 hours after stimulation of the serum-starved cells. The % stimulation was determined relative to stimulation with 5% FBS.
c: wpf = protein fractions obtained from winter-hibernating plasma
d: spf = protein fractions obtained from summer-active plasma
e: Tested fractions are the same as in Table 2.

REFERENCES

1. Wang LCH: Energetic and field aspects of mammalian torpor: The Richardson's ground squirrel. In: Wang LCH, Hudson JW, eds. Strategies in Cold: Natural Torpidity and Thermogenesis. New York: Academic Press, 1978:109-145.

2. Lyman CP, O'Brien RC, Greene GC, Papafrangos ED: Hibernation and longevity in the Turkish hamster Mesocricetus branti. Science 1981; 212:668-670.

3. Barnes BM: Freeze avoidance in a mammal: Body temperature below 0°C in an arctic hibernator. Science 1989; 244:1593-1595.

4. Storey KB: Regulation of liver metabolism by enzyme phosphorylation during mammalian hibernation. J Biol Chem 1987; 262:1670-1673.

5. Riedesel ML, Steffen JM: Protein metabolism and urea recycling in rodent hibernators. Fed Proc 1980; 39:2959-2963.

6. Wolfe RR, Nelson RA, Wolfe MH, Rogers L: Nitrogen cycling in hibernating bears. 30th Annual Conference on Mass Spectrometry and Allied Topics 1982; 426. (Abstract)

7. Kruman II, Kolaeva SG. Iljasova EN, Zubrikhina GN, Khachko VN, Petrova AS: Seasonal variations of DNA synthesis in intestinal epithelial cells of hibernating animals: I. DNA synthesis in intestinal epithelial cells of ground squirrel (*Citellus undulatus*) during hibernation. Comp Biochem Physiol 1986; 83B:173-177.

8. Axelrod LR: Hibernation-a biological timeclock. Prog Biomed Res 1964; 10: 145-151.

9. Swan H, Schatte C: Antimetabolic extract from the brain of the hibernating ground squirrel, *Citellus tridecemlineatus*. Science 1977; 195:84-85.

10. Johansson B: Brown fat: A review. Metabolism 1959; 8:221-240.

11. Popovic V, Vidovic V: Les Glandes surrenales et le sommeil hibernat. Arch Sci Biol 1951; 3:3-17.

12. Pengelley ET, Kelly KH: Plasma potassium and sodium concentrations in active and hibernating golden-mantled ground squirrels, *Citellus lateralis*. Comp Biochem Physiol 1967; 20:299-305.

13. Willis JS, Fang LS, Foster RF: The significance and analysis of membrane function in hibernation. In: Hannon JP, Willis JR, Pengelley EJ, Alpert NR, eds. Hibernation and Hypothermia; Perspectives and Challenges. Ansterdam: Elsevier North Holland, 1972: 123-147.

14. Dawe AR, Spurrier WA: Hibernation induced in ground squirrels by blood transfusion. Science 1969; 163:298-299.

15. Rosser SP, Bruce DS: Induction of summer hibernation in 13-lined ground squirrel *Citellus tridecemlineatus*. Cryobiology 1978; 15:113-116.

16. Tuggy MD, Bruce DC, Pearson PJ: Induction of summer hibernation in 13-lined ground squirrel (*Citellus tridecemlineatus*) by injection of urine or plasma from the bats (*Myotis lucifugus* or *Eptesicus fuscus*). Fed Proc 1983; 42:1254. (Abstract)

17. Bruce DS, Cope GW, Elam TR, Ruit KA, Oeltgen PR, Su TP: Opioids and hibernation. I. Effects of naloxone on bear HIT's depression of guinea pig ileum contractility and on induction of summer hibernation in the ground squirrel. Life Sci 1987; 41:2107-2113.

18. Bruce DS, Darling NK, Seeland KJ, Oeltgen PR, Nilekani SP, Amstrup SC: Is the polar bear (*Ursus Maritimus*) a hibernator? Continued studies on opioids and hibernation. Pharmacol Biochem Behav 1990; 35:705-711.

19. Ruit KA, Bruce DS, Chien PP, Oeltgen PR, Welborn JR, Hilekani SP: Summer hibernation in ground squirrels (*Citellus tridecemlineatus*) induced by injection of whole or fractionated plasma from hibernating black bears (*Ursus americanus*). J Therm Biol 1987; 12:135-138.

20. Oeltgen PR, Bergmann LC, Spurrier WA, Jones SB: Isolation of a hibernation inducing trigger(s) from the plasma of hibernating woodchucks. Prep Biochem 1978; 8:171-188.

21. Oeltgen PR, Spurrier WA: Characterization of a hibernation induction trigger. In: Musacchia XJ, Jansky L, eds. Survival in the Cold: Hibernation and Other Adaptations. New York: Elsevier North Holland, Inc., 1981:139-157.

22. Oeltgen PR, Spurrier WA, Bergmann LC: Hemoglobin alterations of the 13-lined ground squirrel while in various activity states. Comp Biochem Physiol 1979; 64B:207-211.

23. Haglund H: Isoelectric focusing in pH gradients. A technique for fractionation and characterization of ampholytes. Methods Biochem Anal 1971; 19:1-104.

24. Hjalmarsson S: Preparative isotachophoresis-The effect of using ampholine of different pH ranges as spacer ions in the fractionation of serum proteins. Sci Tools 1975; 22:35-38.

25. Travis J, Pannell R: Selective removal of albumin from plasma by affinity chromatography. Clin Chim Acta 1973; 49:49-52.

26. Galster WA, Morrison P: Seasonal changes in serum lipids and proteins in the 13-lined ground squirrel. Comp Biochem Physiol 1966; 18:489-501.

27. Spurrier WA, Dawe AR: Several blood and circulatory changes in the hibernation of the 13-lined ground squirrel, *Citellus tridecemlineatus*. Comp Biochem Physiol 1973; 44A:267-282.

28. Rotermund AJ, Veltman JC: Modification of membrane-bound lipids in erythrocytes of cold-acclimated and hibernating 13-lined ground squirrels. Comp Biochem Physiol 1981; 69B:523-528.

29. Adler MW: Opioid peptides. Life Sci 1980; 26:497-510.

30. Oeltgen PR, Walsh JW, Hamann SR, Randall DC, Spurrier WA, Myers RD: Hibernation "trigger" opioid-like inhibitory action on brain function of the monkey. Pharmacol Biochem Behav 1982; 17:1271-1274.

31. Myers RD, Oeltgen PR, Spurrier WA: Hibernation "trigger" injected in brain induces hypothermia and hypophagia in the monkey. Brain Res Bull 1981; 7:691-695.

32. Meeker RB, Meyers RD, McCalleb ML, Ruwe WD, Oeltgen PR: Suppression of feeding in the monkey by intravenous or cerebroventricular infusion of woodchuck hibernation trigger. Physiologist 1979; 22:86. (Abstract)

33. Oeltgen PR, Blouin RA, Spurrier WA, Myers RD: Hibernation "trigger" alters renal function in the primate. Physiol Behav 1985; 34:79-81.

34. Randall DC, Brady JV, Martin KH: Cardiovascular dynamics during classical apetitive and aversive conditioning in laboratory primates. Pavlov J Biol 1975; 10:66-75.

35. Myers RD: Chronic methods-intraventricular infusion, CSF sampling and push-pull perfusion. In: Myers RD, ed. Methods in psychobiology. Vol 3. New York: Academic Press, 1977: 281-315.

36. Myers RD, Yaksh TL, Hall GH, Veale WL: A method of perfusion of cerebral ventricles of the conscious monkey. J Appl Physiol 1971; 30:589-592.

37. Davis BJ: Disc electrophoresis II: Method and application to human serum proteins. Ann NY Acad Sci 1964; 121:404-427.

38. Chrambach A, Reisfeld RA, Wykoff M, Zaccari J: A procedure for rapid and sensitive staining of protein fractionated by polyacrylamide gel electrophoresis. Anal Biochem 1967; 20:150-154.

39. Margules DL, Goldman B, Finck A: Hibernation: An opioid-dependent state. Brain Res Bull 1979; 4:721-724.

40. Beckman AL, Llados-Edkman S, Stanton TL, Adler MW: Physical dependence on morphine fails to develop during the hibernating state. Science 1981; 212:1527-1529.

41. Hardy JD, Wolff HG, Goodell H: Studies on pain. A new method for measuring pain threshold: Observations on spatial summation of pain. J Clin Invest 1940; 19:649-657.

42. Martin WR, Eades CG, Thompson WO, Thompson JA, Flanary HG: Morphine physical dependence in the dog. J Pharmacol Exp Ther 1974; 189:759-771.

43. Martin WR, Eades CG, Thompson JA, Huppler RE, Gilbert PE: The effects of morphine- and nalorphine-like drugs in the nondependent and morphine-dependent chronic spinal dog. J Pharmacol Exp Therap 1976; 197:517-532.

44. Wettstein JG, Kamerling SG, Martin WR: Effects of microinjection of opioids into and electrical stimulation of the canine periaqueductal gray on EEG electrogenesis, heart rate, pupil diameter, behavior and analgesia. Soc Neurosci Abstr 1982; 8:229-229.

45. Oeltgen PR, Welborn JR, Nuchols PA, Spurrier WA, Bruce DS, Su TP: Opioids and

hibernation. II. Effects of kappa opioid U69593 on induction of hibernation in summer-active ground squirrels by "hibernation induction trigger" (HIT). Life Sci 1987; 41:2115-2120.

46. Su TP, Oeltgen PR, Nuchols PA, Nilekani SP, Spurrier WA: Delta opioid receptor ligand selectively induced hibernation in summer-active ground squirrels. FASEB J 1988; 2:A1074. (Abstract)

47. Oeltgen PR, Nilekani SP, Nuchols PA, Spurrier WA, Su TP: Further studies on opioids and hibernation: delta opioid receptor ligand selectively induced hibernation in summer-active ground squirrels. Life Sci 1988; 43:1565-1574.

48. Turker MS, Monnat RJ, Fukuchi K, et al: A novel class of unstable 6-thioguanine resistant cells from dog and human kidneys. Cell Biol Toxicol 1988; 4:211-223.

49. Pozzatti R, Muschel R, Williams J et al: Primary rat embryo cells transformed by one of two oncogenes show different metastatic potentials. Science 1986; 232:223-227.

50. Balk SD, Levine SP, Young LL, Lafleur MM, Raymond NM: Mitogenic factors present in serum but not in plasma. Proc Natl Acad Sci USA 1981; 78:5656-5660.

51. McNeil PL, McKenna MP, Taylor DL: A transient rise in cytosolic calcium follows stimulation of quiescent cells with growth factors and is inhibitable with phorbol myristate acetate. J Cell Biol 1985; 101:372-379.

CHAPTER 2

DEVELOPMENT OF ORGAN PRESERVATION TECHNIQUES

It is estimated that in the United States as many as 15,000 people die each year who could conceivably benefit from a heart transplant;[1] however, the actual number of people who will benefit is severely constrained by the lack of donor organs. Because of donor age and other contraindications, only 1,000-2,000 viable donor hearts may be available each year.[1,2] This number has been increased somewhat each year as age limits have been extended and as more people become aware of organ donation. However, the plateau of heart and heart-lung transplantation reached after 1987 appears to be primarily related to limited donor availability.[3,4] The criteria for lung donors are even more strict; only 10%-15% of suitable heart donors will also be potential lung donors.[5] Modern technology has made viable tissues (blood cells, cornea, semen, etc.) transfusable or transplantable after years of cryogenic storage,[6] but large organs, such as the heart, lung and liver, can routinely be kept alive for only a few hours prior to transplantation. All large organ transplant procedures must be performed as emergencies.[7,8] Although the recent development of the University of Wisconsin Solution allows the kidney to be preserved for more than 24 hours and the liver to be stored for more than 12 hours,[9] safe preservation of the heart and lungs is still limited to 4-6 hours. The primary cause of death in the first 30 days after heart transplantation remains of cardiac origin rather than from rejection or infection.[3] Increased 30-day mortality correlates with increased ischemic time.[10]

Extended preservation of vital organs, when such a procedure is developed, might have many advantages.

1) It will facilitate transporting organs from donor to recipient and will allow transplantation teams to travel a much longer distance or even worldwide to retrieve and exchange donor organs. Transplantable organs will be transported from one hospital to another, or even from one country to another.[11-19]

2) It will transform transplantation procedures into elective surgery, thus allowing for better preparation of the patients and of the hospital staff and facilities.[6,14-16,20-21]

3) It will facilitate tissue typing by providing more time for matching donors and recipients, a time-consuming process.[6,14-16,21-22]

4) It will help to gain anonymity for the donor, thus reducing undesirable publicity.[21]

5) Finally, it will create an extensive pool of available organs and eliminate the recipient waiting list. Even an organ bank will be made possible.[6,14,20,21]

Although the process is still prospective, true long-term organ preservation will also allow physicians to treat the donor organ and change its antigenicity before it is transplanted, thus reducing or eliminating immunosuppressive treatment of the recipient.[23-28] The ability of the host immunologic system to discriminate the transplanted tissue is another major block in organ transplantation. Studies have shown that the singular presence of histocompatibility complex antigen does not always bring about an immune response leading to graft rejection. However, the presence of interstitial donor "passenger" leukocytes provides the major immunogenic stimulus for the host, resulting in homograft reaction.[23,29-31] The possibility of graft modification has become the subject of extensive research in the past three decades.[23] Three major findings have made graft modification an interesting possibility: 1) the culture conditions of high oxygen concentration are selectively toxic to the vascular bed and to the lymphoreticular elements in the graft, thus permitting nonrecognition by the host and prolonged allograft survival;[23,32-35] 2) lowering the temperature during culture adversely affects the immunogenicity of lymphoreticular cells but not their antigenicity;[23,36-38] 3) pretreatment with radiation, drugs, and donor-specific antibody could alter immunogenicity and reduce rejection.[24,30,39-45] In addition, long periods of organ culture itself could deplete the tissue of viable hematogenous elements and lymphoid cells that could take part in allogenic interactions with host lymphoid cells.[23,46-49]

DEVELOPMENT OF DIFFERENT TECHNIQUES FOR ORGAN PRESERVATION

Successful organ preservation depends upon the balance between metabolic energy requirements, oxygen and nutrient supplies, and the efficacy of the disposal of metabolic waste products. A satisfactory technique for organ preservation must meet four fundamental and interdependent requirements: 1) controlling the metabolism and energy requirements of the organ, 2) administering necessary nutrients, 3) providing the required oxygen, and 4) removing cellular metabolic waste products.[50] Metabolism can be reduced by hypothermia, metabolic inhibitors or freezing of the organ, whereas the circulation can be imitated with perfusion of the organs.[51] All currently used techniques are based on these two basic approaches. Unfortunately, none of the techniques has fulfilled all the requirements for successful organ preservation.

Experiments concerned with preserving the function of organs after their removal from the body for physiologic studies began in the nineteenth century. Numerous studies for developing and improving techniques for organ preservation have been reported. It is impossible to review in detail the historical development of organ preservation in this chapter. Instead, we will review the evolution of different organ preservation techniques, which may shed some light on future improvement and development of new techniques.

MECHANICAL PERFUSION

Mechanical perfusion was the earliest technique used for organ preservation. The idea of artificial perfusion was suggested by Le Gallois in 1812. He mentioned that, by artificial perfusion, life might be kept up in any portion of the animal separated from the rest of the body.[52] In 1828, Kay showed that artificial perfusion with blood was capable of restoring irritability to dying muscle.[52] Artificial perfusion of the kidney was first attempted in 1849 by Lobell.[52] In 1858, Brown-Sequard forced oxygenated blood through an animal's severed head and observed temporary reestablishment of some cortical functions.[52,53] In the 1870s, DeCyon studied the function of an isolated frog's heart perfused with aerated blood for over 24 hours. He also found that an isolated perfused liver was able to manufacture urea.[53,54] Nonblood perfusion of the isolated heart was first reported by Ringers in 1881.[55] He was able to maintain strong heart beats for as long as 4.5 hours using an electrolyte solution that, after subsequent modifications, became known as Ringer's solution. In 1885, von Frey and Gruber devised a special arrangement for continuous aeration of perfusate and for quantitative determination of the blood gas changes in the perfusion.[56]

In the late nineteenth century, various forms of perfusion apparatus were devised by different researchers.[56,57] Because oxygenating blood required mixing air bubbles, which caused difficulties in separation, Jacobj used an isolated lung to oxygenate the blood for heart perfusion, eliminating the direct mixing of blood with the air.[57,58] Langendorff devised a temperature- and pressure-controlled perfusion apparatus which allowed investigation of the mechanical activity of the completely isolated mammalian heart.[59] This method became a standard for subsequent isolated heart function studies. In 1903, Brodie presented his improved design for continuous isolated organ perfusion using autologous blood and glass wool filters during perfusion.[58]

Alexis Carrel was the first person to use various techniques for preserving tissues and organs with transplantation in mind. His transplantation program included the blood vessels, thyroid glands, adrenal glands, parathyroids, ovaries, spleen, intestine, kidneys and several mass transplantations.[60-63] He speculated on the possibility of organ preservation by stating, "It would be important to know whether kidneys extirpated from an animal after a suspension of life of some duration, can resume efficiently their functions."[60] Later on, Carrel reported detailed results of a dog kidney autotransplanted after being flushed with Locke's solution and stored at room temperature for 50 minutes.[64] Carrel won the Nobel Prize in Physiology and Medicine in 1912.[65]

Belt and colleagues brought attention to tissue injury caused by artificial perfusion. They described perfusion injuries including edema, congestion and hemorrhage caused by electrolyte solutions and heterologous blood, and they emphasized the damage to organs caused by warm ischemia prior to the estab-

lishment of perfusion. They emphasized that physiologic perfusion of organs is a matter of great difficulty because solutions containing abnormal quantities of inorganic salts are toxic to the perfused organs.[52] In 1933, Daly and Thorpe used an artificial oxygenator designed by Hooker[66] and Drinker[67] to study heart function and found that the heart quickly became hypodynamic in spite of good oxygenation of the blood; the average duration of heart beat was only 36 minutes. They modified the artificial oxygenator by incorporating two filters, which extended survival time substantially. They pointed out that either the lungs or the filters in the heart-lung preparation were acting as simple mechanical filters of normal or abnormal blood constituents, which if allowed to enter the circulation gradually led to occlusion of the coronary blood vessels. They reemphasized the importance of blood filtration for heart perfusion.[68]

In 1935 Lindbergh developed a perfusion apparatus with which he and Carrel perfused organs for 20-40 days with normothermic serum or synthetic perfusates, demonstrating the viability of some cells by physiologic and histologic studies.[65] They perfused hearts for several days at normothermia with moderate degrees of fiber degeneration and edema. In his classic statement, Carrel set down the requirements for all artificial perfusion, including organ preservation, cardiopulmonary bypass and physiologic studies:

"...the life of the perfused tissues depends on many factors. The fluid must be free of floating particles that may act as emboli. If blood is used, there should be no agglutinated corpuscles. The temperature, the osmotic pressure, the pH of the fluid, the pulse rate, the maximum pressure, the minimum pressure, have to be exactly adjusted. The chemical composition of the nutrient medium and its oxygenation are of capital importance. Moreover, it is imperative that the organ be completely protected against bacteria. Even if all conditions except one are satisfactory, the result of the experiment is utter failure."[69]

Because of the basic anatomic and pathologic differences between human organs and those of the usual laboratory animals, in the 1930s attempts were made to develop a method which would make possible studies on the revived human heart. Kountz achieved the greatest measure of success. In 1936, he used an artificial pump to revive cadaver hearts and was able to restore heart beats for as long as six hours after death. With this technique he studied bundle block, nervous regulations of the heart, coronary flow, and actions of some drugs in human hearts; his results differed from those obtained with animal studies.[70] In the next two decades, perfusion techniques were improved and, in many cases, combined with the use of hypothermia for kidney preservation. In 1951, Lefebvre and Brull reported the results of perfusing dog kidneys with cold saline. After 3-24 hours of storage, they retransplanted the kidneys and were able to re-establish renal function for several hours.[71] In 1954, Murray performed the first successful human kidney transplantation between identical twins.[65,72]

Clinical perfusion techniques developed rapidly between 1955 and 1965 with an emphasis directed toward cardiac surgery; both experimental and clinical applications were found for different organ preservation techniques as well as for postmortem support of organs from donor cadavers.[73-78] In 1958, Couch et al reported the use of simple diluents, including normal saline and Locke's solution in association with blood perfusion for kidney preservation. Bubble oxygenators were also used without passing the blood through a lung at room temperature. Using this technique it was possible to maintain urine production for about seven hours.[79] In 1964, Pegg and Calne reported the use of cooled blood perfusion, which enabled them to autograft two life-sustaining dog kidneys after 24-hours' storage at 0-1°C. Their perfusion with nonsanguinous solution was unsuccessful.[80] In 1963, Humphries and his associates reported successful kidney autotransplantation after 24 hours of continuous hypothermic perfusion with diluted plasma or serum in association with delayed contralateral nephrectomy.[81] The next year, they reported the first successful 24-hour kidney storage combined with immediate contralateral nephrectomy using a pump- membrane oxygenator, a glass wool filter, a low pressure perfusion, hypothermia and diluted autolo-

gous and homologous blood.[82,83] Shorter periods of preservation were also reported by others.[84,85]

In early studies of kidney perfusion, when whole blood was used, a common observation was the onset of marked increases of renal vascular resistance within a few minutes. Consequently, flow through capsular and ureteral collaterals increased visibly, whereas these vessels passed little or no blood initially.[52,73,84-86] Similar events were found with perfusion of the liver. Vascular resistance rose, flow decreased, and the liver trapped blood in large quantities. Many theories were formed to explain the phenomena which resulted in gradual slowing of perfusion flow, including injury to cells[52] and release of vasoactive hormones.[53,75] In 1967, Belzer and his associates reported successful preservation of the kidneys with undiluted plasma under hypothermic pulsatile perfusion for 24 and 72 hours. They retransplanted the preserved kidneys to the donor dog from which the contralateral kidneys had been removed prior to the transplantation.[87,88] The next year, they reported a successful human cadaveric kidney transplantation after 17 hours of preservation.[89] They first eliminated platelet and blood cell aggregates by selecting plasma as the perfusate. Damage to the kidney and rising perfusion pressure were still observed. Conventional microscopic studies showed no evidence of thrombi. However, fat stains revealed multiple microthrombi in the renal arterioles and fat droplets in the tubules and intratubular cells. Belzer and colleagues performed preliminary denaturation of the lipoproteins by freezing and quick thawing, followed by serial filtrations with micropore filters to eliminate the flocculation present in the plasma. In this way, they were able to perfuse dog kidneys for three days without a rise in perfusion pressure. Blockage of the renal arterioles with low-density lipoproteins and deposits of fat droplets in the tubular and intratubular cells had been one of the major causes of previous failure. Since then, although various perfusates are still being tested, cold perfusion with various solutions has gained wide acceptance as a method of short-term organ preservation.[90-97] Successful preservations of dog kidneys and human cadaver kidneys for 4-7 days by pulsatile perfusion, membrane oxygenation, and hypothermia have been reported.[97-99]

Although perfusion preservation was successful for up to 72 hours for the kidney and met with some success for the liver and pancreas,[75,100-105] preservation time for other organs still fell short. In 1969, Feemster and Lillehei reported using a hypothermic-hyperbaric pulsatile perfusion system to preserve canine hearts for 4-24 hours. One dog survived more than eight days after receiving the heart, which had been preserved for 24 hours.[96] In 1972, Martin et al reported their findings concerning a cation transport system in the cell membrane.[106] Researchers began to develop different components for heart and liver preservation. In 1974, using the most modern techniques, including a silica-free, silicone rubber-coated membrane lung, Suaudeau et al were able to maintain strong ventricular activity in sheep hearts for 24-72 hours at 5°-13°C.[107-109] Continuous hypothermic perfusion using crystalloid-based perfusates has experimentally extended successful heart preservation for 24-48 hours.[110-117] Perfusion preservation has also been used for lung preservation, but the results have been disappointing. The anatomic and physiologic peculiarities of the lung, such as its airway system, its low pressure circulation, and the delicate structure of its capillaries facing the alveolar spaces, have raised unique problems.[12,118,119] Methods allowing short-term storage of kidneys, livers, and hearts have not been effective for lung preservation. Although successful preservation for 6-21 hours with blood or crystalloid solutions has been reported,[120-122] continuous normothermic perfusion of isolated lungs with different perfusates usually results in pulmonary edema in a short time.[119,122-124] Normothermic blood perfusion of the isolated dog lung in a special chamber using a support animal as a deoxygenator has maintained pulmonary function and morphology for up to 18 hours. Substitution of a bubble deoxygenator in the system led to rapid functional deterioration after 2-6 hours of perfusion.[121] One reason for failure after lung transplantation is alveolo-capillary block, probably caused by insufficient capillary flow during preservation.[123] At the present time, the safe preservation time for the lungs is still limited to less than six hours,[120] and clinical heart-lung transplantation has been performed only with an on-site donor.[125]

Another type of mechanical perfusion uses whole-body perfusion hypothermia by cardiopulmonary bypass and preserves the organs in situ. The first use of this technique was reported by Starzl and colleagues in 1963. Using this technique in dogs they harvested the kidney and liver at 15°C and then homotransplanted them. The total time from death to revascularization ranged from 2-14.5 hours; the longest survival was 52 days.[78] They also reported three clinical liver transplantations using this technique. Two patients survived 7.5 and 22 days, respectively, but died from pulmonary emboli.[126] Successful use of this technique has been reported by others; one report describes a clinical heart-lung organ block procured 281 minutes away.[125,127-130] Longer periods of preservation time have been reported in animal experiments.[131] This technique offers optimal circumstances for meticulous dissection combined with the abrogation of damaging reflexes associated with hypotension and retraction.[127] It is especially useful for multiorgan harvesting.[128] However, this technique requires both the donor and recipient to be in the same hospital; thus, transportation of either the donor body or the recipient is required.

The essential components of successful kidney perfusion preservation appear to be: 1) hypothermia, 2) a colloid such as albumin to prevent tissue edema, 3) an osmolality of about 300 mOsm/liter obtained with electrolytes, hydrogen ion buffers, and other metabolites, and 4) low perfusion pressure.[132] Many perfusion fluids have been shown to satisfactorily preserve the viability of the kidney for 48-72 hours. Although minor renal damage may occur during the preservation period, the damage is reversible. Attempts to prolong the preservation of kidneys for more than 72 hours have generally achieved inconsistent results. Several reasons contribute to the lack of success of longer storage periods, such as buildup of by-products of metabolic waste, exhaustion of an essential substance in the perfusate, and intrinsic damage to the organ during perfusion.[98,133] For the heart, continuous hypothermic perfusion has extended the ischemic interval to 24 hours or longer in experimental settings.[6,134-136]

The main advantages of continuous perfusion are twofold. First, perfusion provides a continuous supply of oxygen and nutrients for metabolism. Second, metabolic wastes can be removed, eliminating dangerous toxic metabolite buildup. The main drawback of continuous perfusion is the requirement for a perfusion apparatus, which is not only cumbersome but also vulnerable to bacteria contamination. For the heart, a possible disadvantage may be the relative underperfusion of the left ventricle during the perfusion period.[115]

HYPOTHERMIA

Alexis Carrel was one of the first investigators to use hypothermia for tissue storage before transplantation. In his preservation and transplantation experiments, he used hypothermia and freezing techniques to store arteries in Locke's solution for 1-35 days and transplanted them after 10 days of storage. In 1924, Avramovici homografted dog kidneys cooled for periods of up to 30 hours. After removal of the contralateral kidney from an animal, he reported survival of the animal for 36 days.[137] In 1947, Parkinson and Woodworth reported a successful autograft of a seven-day hypothermically preserved goat's kidney without contralateral nephrectomy.[138] The next year, Oudot reported preservation of dog kidneys at $4°C$ for periods of up to eight days followed by homotransplantation, but infarction was found in all kidneys as soon as blood flow was reestablished.[139] Observations in the early 1950s confirmed that hypothermia significantly reduced heart and renal damage resulting from periods of ischemia,[140,141] and considerable effort was directed toward total protection of organ function with various types of regional hypothermia. In the late 1950s and early 1960s, it was well established that reducing the me-

tabolism of the kidney by cooling enabled it to withstand relatively prolonged periods of ischemia. Oxygen consumption decreased exponentially with falling temperature, reaching exceedingly low levels at temperatures within a degree of zero.[74,142] In 1956, Archibald and Cawley autotransplanted dog kidneys that had been cooled to $4°C$ in a saline or dry environment for 24 hours. After autotransplantation, urine was excreted in small amounts and was usually blood-tinged. These kidneys functioned for an average of 7.6 days; the longest survival was 14 days.[143] In 1959, Schloerb et al reported hypothermic kidney storage for up to eight hours by simple cold immersion; survival and restoration of normal renal function was achieved.[55,144] In 1960, Lapchinsky reported detailed results of autografts of 67 canine limbs and 52 kidneys after refrigeration of 24 hours or longer with perfusion at the beginning and end of storage. Using a delayed contralateral nephrectomy, he reported permanent functional survival of 16 dogs for three years and longer.[55] In 1960 and 1961, Kiser et al reported that, after total extracorporeal ischemia of dog kidneys for seven hours, the animal survived on the flushed, refrigerated, and retransplanted kidney for over one year after contralateral nephrectomy.[145,146] Dempster et al reported their results of dog kidney preservation with plasma flushing. The kidneys were placed in normal saline and stored at $4°C$ for six hours. Homotransplantation was performed with moderate success. A clinical kidney transplantation was tried after four hours of storage, but the transplanted organ was rejected within one month.[147] In 1963, Simso et al reported the results of autografting baboon kidneys that had been preserved for 4-22.5 hours by hypothermic storage.[76] Simple cold storage gained popularity in the 1960s for the preservation of the kidney,[147-155] heart,[22,156-159] lungs[160-162] and other organs.[14,53]

Hypothermic storage was further inspired by the observations of Keeler and his colleagues in 1966.[163,164] They perfused rat kidneys with 0.9% sodium chloride at $0°C$ at a pressure of 120 mmHg and found a 50% loss of tissue potassium within 30 minutes and a 16% loss of magnesium over three hours.

There was a concurrent 73% gain in water and a 172% gain in sodium. They concluded that prolonged perfusion of kidneys with physiologic solutions removes essential substances from the cytoplasm but that this loss can be prevented by using solutions containing cations in quantities approaching those normally present in the cells.[163] Using dog kidneys, Martin et al confirmed Keeler's findings and concluded that surface cooling of the canine kidney at 5°C can provide excellent preservation for eight hours. They believed that perfusion offered no advantage for eight-hour storage.[90] In 1969, Collins and associates reported the results of using intracellular crystalloid solutions for hypothermic renal storage. They were able to preserve canine kidneys for 24-30 hours and retransplant them with excellent results.[154] Collins' solutions were continually improved by his group and by others researchers over the subsequent years.[165,166] Studies have confirmed the value of hyperosmolar, hyperkalaemic and hypermagnesaemic flush solutions for the storage of rabbit, pig, dog and human kidneys for periods of up to 72 hours.[164]

The simplicity of hypothermic storage stimulated other researchers to use this technique as an alternative to perfusion for transplantation. In 1973, Sacks et al reported their results of an improved hyperosmolar intracellular solution for kidney preservation for up to 72 hours after initial perfusion and hypothermic storage.[92] The first clinical long-distance heart procurement was reported by Thomas and colleagues in 1978. They traveled as far as 1400 km with a total ischemic time of 3 hours 15 minutes. The patient did well after surgery.[167] In 1979, Toledo-Pereyra et al reported their results of preserving pancreas allografts in a colloid hyperosmolar solution for 48 hours.[168] In 1981, Squifflet et al reported their use of Euro-Collins solution to preserve human cadaver kidneys. After transplantation, postoperative survival and renal function demonstrated that up to 51 hours of preservation was safe.[169] Studies at that time indicated that cold storage was successful for human kidneys for up to 24-50 hours.[169,170]

The improvement of modern hypothermic storage should be credited to Dr. Belzer at the University of Wisconsin. His group did meticulous research with tissue slices and whole organs. He found the biochemical differences between the kidney, the liver, and the pancreas in cell swelling and enzyme activity. Based on his observations, he designed a solution that was not only appropriate for the cold storage of the kidney but also successful for storing the pancreas and the liver.[9] The solution was tested in the preservation of the dog pancreas, and for the first time successful and consistent 72-hour preservation was obtained.[171] Currently, flushing solutions using hypothermia are most effective for kidney preservation. If a kidney is placed in ice-cold saline immediately after its removal and kept at 0°-4°C, little deterioration occurs in up to 8 hours of storage.[26] According to Schirmer and Walton, hypothermia reduces the oxygen consumption of renal cortex to 1/3 at 27°C, to 1/6 at 17°C, and to almost zero at 7°C.[155] The reduction of metabolism is relatively more severe in the kidney than are the changes for the whole body at equivalent temperatures.[172] The effectiveness of this solution for other organs is under extensive investigation. According to Belzer et al, the normal intracellular concentrations of sodium and potassium are maintained by an energy-dependent cation transport system in the cell membrane. Although this system is a universal component of cellular tissues, kidney tissue possesses greater ATPase activity at normothermia than does either heart or liver. Hypothermia depresses ATPase activity in tissues so that sodium and water enter the cell and potassium moves out. At 10°C, the kidney is the only organ in which the energy-dependent cation transport system is active, a situation which does not hold for the heart or liver.[106] Reported experimental effective lung preservation times using different solutions vary widely, ranging from several hours[12,173-183] to several days.[184-188] However, safe clinical preservation time is still limited to less than six hours.[189] Currently, the UW solution, the modified Collins solution, the UCLA solution, and other formulas are under extensive investigation for further improvement and possible use in the preservation of other organs.[9,112,182,190-195]

Among all the methods used, hypothermic storage is the simplest and least expensive method of preservation. Hypothermia exerts a marked depression on the rate of oxidative metabolism. Cooling can arrest the rapid deterioration that occurs in an organ at 37°C when deprived of its blood supply. We can speculate that the present hypothermic storage time is likely to be increased further and that the number of preservable organs will be expanded when more effective preservation solutions are developed. Hypothermic storage has two major limitations. First, substrates for metabolism are not provided, and a collapsed, blocked microcirculation may remain so until the organ is transplanted, which could result in tissue damage.[196] Second, metabolism is not completely suppressed by temperatures above 0°C, even in the presence of chemical metabolic inhibitors. Significant active transport persists even at 0°C.[15,157,165] If organs are kept at 0°-4°C, although metabolism is reduced, oxygen consumption is still approximately 5% of normal. It is not possible to cool the heart sufficiently to permit prolonged storage without freezing it.[157] Hypothermia itself also has adverse effects on cell physiology.[26,164,197] Under hypothermia, the ATPase activity is reduced, which in turn alters the sodium pump activity necessary to maintain normal extracellular and intracellular ion distribution.[106] The intracellular potassium concentration is decreased, and the membrane potential disappears.[198] Chloride ions consequently enter the cell. The intracellular osmotic concentration increases, water streams into the cell, and the cell swells.[199] After the organ is transplanted, this cell swelling prevents normal blood circulation in capillaries and minor blood vessels, resulting in the so-called "no reflow" phenomenon.[51]

Hyperbaria

Attempts have been made to improve the results of hypothermic storage by additional hyperbaric oxygenation. This work gained much attention in the 1960s. Ackermann and Barnard used different combinations of low temperature, perfusion, and hyperbaria to preserve dog kidneys. Only the kidneys preserved at 5°-10°C with 3 atm hyperbaric

oxygen survived transplantation with immediate or delayed contralateral nephrectomy.[200] Researchers in Lillehei's laboratory reported good survival rates when canine kidneys were removed, cooled immediately by perfusion with cold 5% dextran 40 in 0.9% saline solution, stored at 0°-4°C for 24 hours in 100% oxygen at 3 atm pressure, and reimplanted autoplastically with delay of contralateral nephrectomy for 1-4 weeks.[151,152,201] Similar results were obtained for experimental heart and other organ preservations[96,149,150,157,160,202] and for clinical cadaver or living donor renal transplantation.[203] In Tayor's study, high pressure was used for brief periods to accelerate phase transitions during the freezing and thawing of cell suspensions. Cellular damage by pressure was confirmed: the number of cells killed without freezing was proportional to pressure and to the time of exposure. Survival of chick skin cells ranged from 100% at 15,000 psi for three seconds to 0.01% at 35,000 psi for 120 seconds.[204] There is universal agreement that, when cells or tissues are exposed to oxygen pressures in excess of 1 atmosphere, inhibition of tissue metabolism results. The reason for the depression of oxygen consumption is probably related to the inactivation of certain enzyme systems, notably pyruvate oxidase, by high tensions of oxygen. This inhibition may be beneficial in an organ devoid of circulation.[129,205] It is also well known that the freezing point is depressed under increased pressure. However, the freezing point of water is lowered by only 1°C when the pressure over it is increased by 10 atmospheres, so that at 30,000 lbs/in² the freezing point is -20°C. Although red blood cells can withstand pressures of 50,000 lbs/in² at room temperature, whether organs can withstand pressure much greater than 3 atmospheres at close to their freezing temperature is questionable and currently unsolved.[157] Using hyperbaria alone does not work because a pressure of 50 atm must be applied to sufficiently supply the inside of the kidney with oxygen;[202] however, a pressure of that magnitude is toxic for the outer layers of the kidney.[51] Lower oxygen pressure may be sufficient to supply the lungs. More than 4 atm of oxygen pressure at a temperature of 2°-4°C causes irreversible canine lung damage.[206] Due to the complex setup and the uncertainty involved in organ preservation, the hyperbaric oxygenation technique has now been totally replaced by simple hypothermia.

CRYOPRESERVATION

The attraction for further lowering of temperature lies in the possibility of arresting, not merely retarding, chemical reactions, which will lead to indefinite low-temperature banking of organs. In view of the success of prolonged viable preservation of spermatozoa, blood cells and corneas in liquid nitrogen, an effort was made to apply similar techniques to organ conservation in the late 1950s and early 1960s.[156] Smith reported freezing a hamster heart to -20°C and successfully resuscitating it after thawing.[207] In several other studies, animal hearts could be cooled to -2°C to -20°C in the presence of cryoprotective agents (glycerol or dimethyl-sulfoxide), but functional recovery was usually poor and varied widely.[156,158,208,209] In kidney preservation studies, dog kidneys were perfused and cooled to -20°C to -80°C, thawed and reimplanted; some kidneys recovered their function and a few survived for lengthy periods.[210-214] However, such successful preservation has been rare.[213,215]

Factors such as organ geometry, mixed cell types, packing density and cell architecture make it difficult to optimize freezing and thawing rates, and optimal temperatures for individual cells and organs vary substantially.[216,217] Ice formation during cooling and rewarming causes severe cell damage.[218] Isolated parenchymal organs, which require implantation by vascular anastomosis for revival, do not survive the freeze-thaw cycle under present experimental methods, even with the presence of cryophylactic chemical agents.[53,219,220] Vascular endothelial cells, especially the capillaries, are extremely sensitive to low temperatures. The preserved organ becomes rapidly edematous from fluid leaks due to damage to the vascular compartment, which leads to high resistance and eventually stoppage of the circulation.[196,213] On the other hand, freezing alone does not appear to provide the conditions necessary for truly long-term storage. Even when tissues and organisms are "frozen solid" at a few degrees below freezing, deterioration can still occur.[53] Apparently physical, chemical and even biologic activities are still in progress at temperatures well below zero.[53] The cryoprotective agents, in particular glycerol and dimethyl sulfoxide, are difficult to perfuse into the tissues and even more difficult to remove. They also seem to have a toxic effect on some tissues, especially in high concentrations.[26,53]

Researchers have also explored techniques for solidifying organs without freezing-vitrification. High concentrations of cryoprotective agents can solidify into an amorphous state when cooled to a very low temperature. At this point, metabolism is stopped but no ice formation occurs.[214,221,222] This work has not been pursued extensively, and more research is needed.

PARABIOSIS

The living host is obviously the best perfusion apparatus in existence. From the nutritional standpoint, blood remains the ideal perfusate.[53] The concept of interim parabiotic perfusion, requiring the use of a host to perfuse the heart as a mean of preservation, was first introduced by Marcus and coworkers in 1953. They transplanted dog hearts and heart-lungs after preservation with maximum survival times of as long as 44 hours.[223] Their technique involved connecting the host animal's femoral artery to the organ artery. The venous flow returning from the organ went back directly to the host femoral vein[224] or through a pump,[225,226] or it could be used to bathe the organ in a sealed chamber.[77]

In 1965, Gilsdorf et al reported a venous pressure-regulated device for preserving canine kidneys for more than 24 hours. Their dogs survived well on the perfused kidneys.[225] Shumway and associates reported the use of this technique to preserve dog hearts for three days and then transplant them successfully.[227]

Using a living perfusion animal has many advantages. It provides an ideal whole blood perfusate and allows the lung and liver to detoxify vaso-constrictor substances.[86,225,228] With care, the host may be transportable in both experimental and clinical applications. The function of the preserved organ can be assessed during storage. However, regional or whole-body heparinization is necessary. Artificial tubing is still needed for connecting the host and organs.[224] Infection can develop during the preservation period. All of these difficulties could pose some danger to the host.

AUTOPERFUSION

Using an animal's own heart as a pump provides the most convenient setup for physiologic studies, and the animal's own blood provides the best perfusion medium. As far back as 1881, Martin attempted to study the activity of the heart by diverting all the blood from the aorta back into the right atrium, creating a heart-lung preparation. This procedure and its modifications have been used by many researchers. In 1912, Knowlton and Starling reported their modification of Martin's preparation for isolated heart and lung perfusion used for studies of heart function.[229] In 1914, Bainbridge and Evans connected an isolated kidney to Starling's heart-lung preparation to form a heart-lung-kidney preparation for renal function studies.[230] This technique was carried further with the use of two sets of heart-lung-kidney settings for comparison of kidney functions.[231] These preparations closely approached natural conditions.[230] In 1948, the Russian scientist Demikhov used an autoperfused heart-lung perfusion for transplantation.[21] Sen et al attempted to use this technique for preservation purposes in 1956.[232] With the animal at a low rectal temperature ($26°C$), they isolated dog hearts and lungs while they were still perfused by the heart and oxygenated by the lungs. The preparations remained viable for from nine minutes to one hour, too short a time for practical usage. They realized that their system was extremely unbalanced, but they believed that it might be useful for heart-lung transplantation in the future. In 1957, Webb and Howard reported using this technique as a bridge for heart and lung transplantation. Although the dogs were unable to resume spontaneous breathing after lung transplantation, the heart did regain function after transplantation.[233]

Since 1959, autoperfusion has gained more attention for use in organ preservation.

In 1963, Robicsek et al reported an improved heart-lung preparation in which a buffer bag was incorporated into the system so that the blood from the left ventricle had a larger exit, thus reducing the afterload on the left ventricle.[234] The preparation underwent many modifications; finally, a relatively fixed setup was used. The buffer bag was connected to the ascending aorta, and the blood return tubing was connected to the superior vena cava. The blood circulation in the buffer bag was parallel to the coronary system, and survival time was increased.[235] In 1967, Whiffen et al used a similar preparation that connected the heart and left lung for short-term preservation before orthotopic transplantation in dogs.[236] Researchers in Shumway's laboratory extended the study to resuscitation-preservation-transplantation experiments. The hearts were anoxic at $37°C$ for 1-1/2 hours and were preserved in an autoperfusion heart-lung preparation for 6-30 hours. Ten hearts were orthotopically transplanted and were able to take over the circulatory load after bypass for up to 38 hours.[237] Early studies indicated that the preparation suffered several problems, such as progressive metabolic deterioration after 6-12 hours of perfusion, elevation of creatinine phosphokinase and lactate-pyruvate ratio, loss of membrane integrity, continuous bleeding caused by heparinization, and early lung deterioration.[18,235,238-245] The survival time could be increased by extracorporeal symbiosis,[237,241] substrate enhancement,[246] complement inhibitor and platelet depletion,[247] isoproterenol and other drugs.[248,249] At the same time, other researchers used a heart-lung preparation without a buffer bag[18,21,250] and obtained longer survival times than those obtained by Sen et al.[232] In 1987, Hardesty et al used the preparation for successful clinical heart transplantation.[7,251,252] It was generally agreed that this technique was effective for heart preservation up to six hours.[7,243,253]

The main problems with the heart-lung preparation appear to be related to three inherent deficiencies. First, because of the existence of a plastic bag and tubing in the circulation, anticoagulants are always necessary to prevent clotting. Using these agents leads to uncontrollable bleeding after the operation. Second, the foreign material and blood-gas interface cause severe hemolysis. Free plasma hemoglobin has been reported to increase 20-fold within 8 hours.[235,238] Finally, although fluid and nutrients can be added, excessive water and metabolic wastes cannot be removed. Progressive metabolic deterioration occurs 6-12 hours after perfusion starts.[235,238,243,254] This change is not due to lack of available oxygen in the blood,[18,238] but it is a major limiting factor in long-term preservation.[235,238,248,255] Probably the greatest limiting factor of the heart-lung preparation is the early deterioration of the lungs. Even though preservation of the heart is successful for more than 12 hours, the lungs deteriorate quickly and usually become unusable after 4-6 hours of preservation.[46,242,256,257] Numerous spots of subpleural hemorrhage occur early in the preservation, and their size increases with time. Small spots gradually merge together later on and become hemorrhagic blotches. The lungs gradually become stiff and sink in the water bath. Thousands of milliliters of fluid can be excreted from the lungs, and the experiment usually ends with severe lung damage. The results in our laboratory have shown that the blood returning from the buffer bag carries many microthrombi, which are trapped in the lungs during the preservation period. This is probably one of the major causes for early lung deterioration.

Our own interests in autoperfusion started in 1985. We used the heart-lung autoperfusion preparation for heart and lung preservation. The early failure of the lungs during preservation led us to search for the reasons for the different results observed between the heart and lungs in this preparation. Incorporation of a filter in the venous return line demonstrated substantial microthrombi in the filter. This finding reminded us of the complications encountered in the early period of heart-lung bypass. The foreign material in the circulation inevitably introduces platelet and leucocyte aggregation, protein denaturation and microdrops of circulating fat. Although lung damage during preservation could be caused by other factors, elimination of foreign material from the circulation would

increase survival time. A multiorgan preparation without foreign material and blood-gas interfaces was developed.[258] In this preparation, the heart and lungs are removed along with the liver, pancreas, duodenum and both kidneys while they are still perfused by the heart and oxygenated by the lungs. The technique does not induce ischemia during harvesting and preservation. The organs become a self-contained block with a relatively complete physiologic environment. The heart pumps blood; the lungs oxygenate blood. Metabolic wastes are removed; water and electrolyte balance is maintained by the kidneys. Major biochemical processes are performed by the liver. Oxygen, nutrients, electrolytes and antibiotics are continuously supplied to the preparation. The system maintains its natural anatomic connections and physiologic relationship. In our preliminary studies, the survival time has reached more than two days with excellent lung preservation.[259-262]

In contrast to other techniques used so far, this technique appears to preserve all the organs uniformly. We are especially encouraged by the good quality of the lungs. Although many of our preliminary experiments are performed under semisterile or nonsterile conditions, the lungs are still in very good condition after more than 24 hours of preservation. In six experiments, the organs were preserved for 24-33 hours, and the left lungs were removed from the organ blocks and transplanted into six recipients. The opposite pulmonary artery was ligated 0-6 hours postoperatively. Lung function was very good as seen in Chapter 4. We believe this time could be extended further if totally sterile surgery were performed.

This technique also provides several features that cannot be found in other techniques. First, it eliminates ischemic time during organ harvesting. This ischemic time is unavoidable when other techniques such as hypothermia or mechanical perfusion are used. Nonstop circulation during harvesting is especially important for those organs that are sensitive to ischemic damage, such as the lungs, the liver, and, of course, the brain. Second, it provides the most natural physiologic environment. Temperature and blood components can be maintained at physiologic levels as required, any infusion can be given at any time during the perfusion period and toxic metabolites are continuously removed or detoxified. Third, it allows continuous monitoring and studying of organ function during the preservation period. This feature is especially important for such vital organs as the heart and lungs, for which immediate functioning following transplantation is mandatory.

This technique has several drawbacks, however. First, it requires a well-trained operating team to retrieve the organs. Exposing the lung for a long period of time would reduce its preservation time. Second, the organ block is relatively bulky and transportation is more difficult than for a single organ. Third, unlike hypothermic storage, in which the organ can be ignored after it is placed in a refrigerator, the autoperfusion block requires continuous monitoring and appropriate adjustments. However, the technique seems to meet all the fundamental requirements for successful organ preservation. It also provides the most natural physiologic environment for the organs and makes very possible the concept of long-term preservation and organ banks.

Summary

Over the past 40 years, much progress has been made in organ transplantation. Progress in preservation has been slow. Despite the extension of preservation time for the kidneys, safe preservation time for the heart and lungs is still short and has not been increased appreciably since 1959.[263] Clinical studies have demonstrated that ischemic times of more than five hours lead to early heart failure after transplantation.[167,182,264,265] In the study by Lurie et al in 1982, hypothermic storage of rat hearts for up to 12 hours was followed by heterotopic transplantation. Although all hearts functioned well after transplantation, ultrastructural analysis showed that chronic fibrosis occurred in the hearts 50 days after transplantation when the hearts were hypothermically preserved in cardioplegia for more than four hours.[266] A number of other studies have also demonstrated that adequate myocardial preservation is limited to 6-8 hours using presently employed solutions.[167,267]

The difficulties involved in long-term preservation can be seen by the lack of clear definition of "long-term". Studies claiming to have obtained "long-term" survival report times ranging from a few hours[268-270] to less than one day[111,156,267,271,272] to several days.[9,17,273] Until we are able to successfully preserve the organs for at least several days, we cannot do much to dramatically change transplantation procedures. Objective recognition of the advantages and disadvantages of a new technique is only achieved when the technique has been studied extensively. Until then, we can predict some but not all of its potential problems. The artificial heart was believed to be the dream of heart substitutes. However, once it began to be used, the problems encountered were enormous and even today are far from being resolved.

Most of our existing information on organ preservation comes from studies of the kidney. The kidney, a paired organ of small size, considerable reserve and high ability to regenerate, has been the most suitable organ for preservation-transplantation studies. Although it may not be totally safe to generalize from kidney studies to the preservation of other organs, the knowledge gained from kidney preservation provides a base of information for studying preservation techniques for other organs.[274] Future prospects for the advancement in organ preservation lie in a more complete understanding of the nature of hypoxic damage to the organs, in methods that avoid or reduce this kind of damage, and in a more complete understanding of the specific metabolic demands and physiologic requirements of different organs. Further extension in hypothermic storage or mechanical perfusion would require new techniques or new solutions specifically designed for individual organs, as experimental studies have demonstrated.[195] Such studies will require large investments of time and energy. Dr. Hume's statement, made 20 years ago, is still valid today and probably will still be valid 20 years from now: "It would be extremely valuable to have some sort of a kidney bank where kidneys could be stored for many months; however, it looks as though we are a long way from this at the present time."[81]

References

1. Evans RW, Manninen DL, Gersh BJ, Hart LG, Rodin J: The need for and supply of donor hearts for transplantation. J Heart Transplant 1984; 4:57-62.

2. Evans RW, Manninen DL, Garrison LPJr, Maier AM: Donor availability as the primary determinant of the future of heart transplantation. JAMA 1986; 255:1892-1898.

3. Kriett JM, Kaye MP: The registry of the International Society for Heart Transplantation: Seventh official report-1990. J Heart Lung Transplant 1990; 9:323-330.

4. Kriett JM, Kaye MP: The registry of the International Society for Heart and Lung Transplantation: Eighth official report-1991. J Heart Lung Transplant 1991; 10:491-498.

5. Smyth RL, Higenbottam TW, Scott JP, Wallwork J: Transplantation of the lungs. Respir Med 1989; 83:459-466.

6. Armitage WJ: Heart. In: Karow AMJr, Pegg DE, eds. Organ Preservation for Transplantation. 2nd ed. New York: Marcel Dekker, Inc., 1981:577-597.

7. Hardesty RL, Griffith BP: Autoperfusion of the heart and lungs for preservation during distant procurement. J Thorac Cardiovasc Surg 1987; 93:11-18.

8. McMaster P: Techniques of multiple organ harvesting. In: Morris PJ, Tilney NL, eds. Progress in Transplantation. New York: Churchill Livingstone, 1984:209-221.

9. Belzer FO: Principles of organ preservation. Transplant Proc 1988; 20 (suppl 1):925-927.

10. Heck CF, Shumway SJ, Kaye MP: The registry of the International Society for Heart Transplantation: sixth official report-1989. J Heart Transplant 1989; 8:271-276.

11. Editorial:: Moving donors. Nature 1969; 221:9.

12. Keshavjee SH, Yamazaki F, Cardoso PF, McRitchie DI, Patterson GA, Cooper JD: A method for safe 12-hour pulmonary preservation. J Thorac Cardiovasc Surg 1989; 98:529-534.

13. Lim SML, Soh P, Pwee HS, Vathsala A, Rauff A, Foong WC: Trans-Pacific sharing of kidneys requiring preservation for more than 50 hours: an analysis of 33 cases. Transplant Proc 1990; 22:336-337.

14. Marshall VC: Organ preservation. In: Calne RY, ed. Clinical organ transplantation. Oxford:Blackwell Scientific Pub., 1971:55-103.

15. Karow AM Jr: The organ bank concept. In: Karow AMJr, Pegg DE, eds. Organ Preservation for Transplantation. 2nd ed. New York: Marcel Dekker,Inc., 1981:3-12.

16. Southard JH, Belzer FO: Organ preservation. In: Flye MW, ed. Principles of Organ Transplantation. Philadelphia: W.B.Saunders Co., 1989:194-215.

17. Southard JH: Advances in organ preservation. Transplant Proc 1989; 21:1195-1196.

18. Cooper DKC: The donor heart: the present position with regard to resuscitation, storage and assessment of viability. J Surg Res 1976; 21:363-381.

19. Billingham ME, Baumgartner WA, Watson DC, et al: Distant heart procurement for human transplantation: Ultrastructural studies. Circulation 1980; 62 (Suppl. I):11-19.

20. Turner MD: Organ storage. In: Hardy JD, ed. Human Organ Support and Replacement. Springfield: C. C. Thomas Pub., 1971:35-65.

21. Cooper DKC: Haemodynamic studies during short-term preservation of the autoperfusion heart-lung preparation. Cardiovasc Res 1975; 9:753-763.

22. Proctor E, Matthews G, Archibald J: Acute orthotopic transplantation of hearts stored for 72 hours. Thorax 1971; 26:99-102.

23. Hardy MA, Lau HT: Graft modification. In: Flye MW, ed. Principles of Organ Transplantation. Philadelphia: W.B.Saunders Co., 1989:72-90.

24. Guttmann RD, Beaudoin JG, Morehouse DD: Reduction of immunogenicity of human cadaver renal allografts by donor pretreatment. Transplant Proc 1973; 5:663-665.

25. Bretscher P, Cohn M: A theory of self-nonself discrimination. Science 1970; 169:1042-1049.

26. Calne RY: Organ grafts. 1st ed. Baltimore: The Williams & Wilkins Co., 1975.31-37.

27. Belzer FO, Park HY, Vetto RM: Factors influencing renal blood flow during isolated perfusion. Surg Forum 1964; 15:222-224.

28. Collins G: Organ transplantation: the role of preservation. In: Pegg DE, Karow AMJr, eds. The Biophysics of Organ Cryopreservation. New York: Plenum Press, 1987:3-14.

29. Montefusco CM, Veith FJ: Lung transplanta-

tion. In: Flye MW, ed. Principles of Organ Transplantation. Philadelphia: W.B. Saunders Co., 1989:413-435.

30. Lacy PE, Davie JM, Finke EH: Induction of rejection of successful allografts of rat islets by donor peritoneal exudate cells. Transplantation 1979; 28:415-420.

31. Lafferty KJ, Prowse SJ, Simeonovic CJ, Warren HS: Immunobiology of tissue transplantation: a return to the passenger leukocyte concept. Ann Rev Immunol 1983; 1:143-173.

32. Naji A, Silvers WK, Barker CF: Effect of culture in 95% oxygen on the survival of parathyroid allografts. Surg Forum 1979; 30:109-111.

33. Hullett DA, Landry AS, Leonard DK, Sollinger HW: Enhancement of thyroid allograft survival following organ culture: Alteration of tissue immunogenicity. Transplantation 1989; 47:24-27.

34. Talmage DW, Dart GA: Effect of oxygen pressure during culture on survival of mouse thyroid allografts. Science 1978; 200:1066-1067.

35. La Rosa FG, Talmage DW: The failure of a major histocompatibility antigen to stimulate a thyroid allograft reaction after culture in oxygen. J Exp Med 1983; 157:898-906.

36. Opels G, Terasaki PI: Lymphocyte antigenicity loss with retention of responsiveness. Science 1974; 184:464-466.

37. Lacy PE, Davie JM, Finke EH: Prolongation of islet allograft survival following in vitro culture (24°C) and a single injection of ALS. Science 1979; 204:312-313.

38. Abouna GM, Heil JE, Sutherland DER, Najarian JS: Factors necessary for successful 48-hour preservation of pancreas grafts. Transplantation 1988; 45:270-274.

39. Faustman DL, Steinman RM, Gebel HM, Hauptfeld V, Davie JM, Lacy PE: Prevention of rejection of murine islet allografts by pretreatment with antidendritic cell antibody. Proc Natl Acad Sci USA 1984; 81:3864-3868.

40. Ready AR, Jenkinson EJ, Kingston R, Owen JJT: Successful transplantation across major histocompatibility barrier of dioxyguanosine-treated embryonic thymus expressing class II antigens. Nature 1984; 310:231-233.

41. Faustman DL, Steinman RM, Gebel HM, Hauptfeld V, Davie JM, Lacy PE: Prevention of mouse islet allograft rejection by elimination of intraislet dendritic cells. Transplant Proc 1985; 17:420-422.

42. Nowygrod R, Hardy MA, Todd GJ, Oluwole S, Reemtsma K: Donor pretreatment in cardiac allografts. Transplant Proc 1979; 11:1462-1464.

43. Todd GJ, Nowygrod R, Hardy MA, Reemtsma K: Donor and donor organ pretreatment in cardiac allografts. Surg Forum 1978; 29:362-364.

44. Anderson CB, Jendrisak MD, Flye JMW et al. Renal allograft recipient immunomodulation by concomitant immunosuppression and donor-specific transfusions. Transplant Proc 1988; 20:1074-1078.

45. Gough IR, Finnimore M: Rat parathyroid transplantation: Allograft pretreatment with organ culture and antilymphocyte serum. Transplant 1980; 29:149-152.

46. Caspi J, Herman SL, Wilson GJ, et al: Neonatal autoperfused working heart-lung preparation: assessment of factors determining survival. J Heart Transplant 1990; 9:435-440.

47. Sollinger HW, Burkholder PM, Rasmus WR, Bach FH: Prolonged survival of xenografts after organ culture. Surg 1977; 81:74-79.

48. Parr EL, Bowen KM, Lafferty KJ: Cellular changes in cultured mouse thyroid glands and islets of Langerhans. Transplantation 1980; 30:135-141.

49. Lafferty KJ, Bootes A, Dart G, Talmage DW: Effect of organ culture on the survival of thyroid allografts in mice. Transplantation 1976; 22:138-149.

50. Galletti G: Hypothermia and hibernation. In: Karow AMJr, Pegg DE, eds. Organ Preservation for Transplantation. 2nd ed. New York: Marcel Dekker, Inc., 1981:101-111.

51. Grundmann R: Fundamentals of preservation methods. In: Toledo-Pereyra LH, ed. Basic Concepts of Organ Procurement, Perfusion, and Preservation for transplantation. New York: Academic Press, 1982:93-120.

52. Belt AE, Smith HP, Whipple GH: Factors concerned in the perfusion of living organs and tissues. Am J Physiol 1920; 52:101-120.

53. Robertson R, Jacob SW: The preservation of intact organs. Adv Surg 1968; 3:75-159.

54. Toledo-Pereyra LH: Organ preservation I. Kidney and pancreas. J Surg Res 1981; 30:165-180.

55. Lapchinsky AG: Recent results of experimental transplantation of preserved limbs and kidneys and possible use of this technique in clinical practice. Ann NY Acad Sci 1960; 87:539-571.

56. von Frey M, Gruber M: Untersuchungen uber den stoffwechsel isolirter organe I. Ein respirationsapparat fur isolirte organe. Arch Anat Physiol (Leipzig). 1885; 519-532.

57. Jacobj C: Ein Beitrag zur technik der kunstlichen durchblutung uberlebender organe. Arch Exp Pathol Pharmacol. 1895; 36:330-348.

58. Brodie TG: The perfusion of surviving organs. J Physiol (London) 1903; 29:266-275.

59. Doring HJ and Dehnert H: The isolated perfused heart according to Langendorff. March, West Germany: Biomesstechnik-Verlag, 1987.1-16.

60. Carrel A: Transplantation in mass of the kidneys. J Exp Med 1908; 10:98-143.

61. Carrel A: Calcification of the arterial system in a cat with transplanted kidneys. J Exp Med 1908; 10:276-282.

62. Carrel A: Results of the transplantation of blood vessels, organs and limbs. JAMA 1908; 51:1662-1667.

63. Carrel A: On the permanent life of tissues outside of the organism. J Exp Med 1912; 15:516-528.

64. Carrel A: The ultimate result of a double nephrectomy and the replantation of one kidney. J Exp Med 1911; 14:124-125.

65. Humphries AL, Dennis AJ: Historical developments in preservation. In: Toledo-Pereyra LH, ed. Basic Concept of Organ Procurement, Perfusion, and Preservation for Transplantation. New York: Academic Press, 1982:1-30.

66. Hooker DR: The perfusion of the mammalian medulla: the effect of calcium and of potassium on the respiratory and cardiac centers. Am J Physiol 1915; 38:200-208.

67. Drinker CK, Drinker KR, Lund CC: The circulation in the mammalian bone-marrow. Am J Physiol 1922; 62:1-92.

68. Daly IB, Thorpe WV: An isolated mammalian heart preparation capable of performing work for prolonged periods. J Physiol (London) 1933; 79:199-217.

69. Carrel A and Lindbergh CA: The culture of organs. New York: Paul B. Hoeber, 1938.

70. Kountz WB: Revival of human hearts. Ann Intern Med 1936; 10:330-336.

71. Lefebvre L, Brull L: Reins au cou prealablement perfuses et conserves a basse temperature. Compt Rend Seanc (Par) 1951; 145:1895-1899.

72. Murray JE, Merrill JP, Harrison JH: Renal homotransplantation in identical twins. Surg Forum 1955; 6:432-436.

73. Cassie GF, Couch NP, Dammin GJ, Murray JE: Normothermic perfusion and replantation of the excised dog kidney. SGO 1959; 109:721-728.

74. Semb G, Krog J, Johansen K: Renal metabolism and blood flow during local hypothermia, studied by means of renal perfusion in situ. Acta Chir Scand Suppl 1960; 253:196-202.

75. Kestens PJ, Farrelly JA, McDermott WV: A technique of isolation and perfusion of the canine liver. J Surg Res 1961; 1:58-63.

76. Simso LA, Telander RL, Hitchcock CR: Hypertension following renal autografting in the Kenya baboon. Surg Forum 1963; 14:170-171.

77. Zangheri EO, Campana H, Ponce F, Silva JC, Fernandez FO, Suarez JRE: Production of erythropoietin by anoxic perfusion of the isolated kidney of a dog. Nature 1963; 199:572-573.

78. Marchioro TL, Huntley RT, Waddell WR, Starzl TE: Extracorporeal perfusion for obtaining postmortem homografts. Surgery 1963; 54:900-911.

79. Couch NP, Cassie GF, Murray JE: Survival of the excised dog kidney perfused in a pump-oxygenator system. Surgery 1958; 44:666-682.

80. Pegg DE, Calne RY, Pryse-Davies J, Brown FL: Canine renal preservation using surface and perfusion cooling techniques. Ann NY Acad Sci 1964; 120:506-523.

81. Humphries AL, Russell R, Ostafin J, Goodrich SM, Moretz WH: Successful reimplantation of canine kidney after 24 hour storage. Surgery 1963; 54:136-143.

82. Humphries AL, Moretz WH, Peirce EC:

Twenty-four hour kidney storage with report of a successful canine autotransplant after total nephrectomy. Surgery 1964; 55:524-530.

83. Humphries AL, Russell R, Christopher PE, Goodrich SM, Stoddard LD, Moretz WH: Successful reimplantation of twenty-four-hour stored kidney to nephrectomized dog. Ann NY Acad Sci 1964; 120:496-505.

84. Steyn BJ, Mobley TL, Suwanagul A: Factors influencing extracorporeal hypothermic perfusion of the isolated canine kidney. Br J Urol 1966; 38:657-663.

85. Kane JF, Edwards EC: Renal vascular shutdown during perfusion of the isolated kidney. Br J Urol 1966; 38:664-672.

86. O'Connor WJ, Verney EB, Vogt M: The vasoconstrictor activity acquired by defibrinated blood during perfusion of the isolated kidney of the dog. Q J Exp Physiol 1941; 31:1-24.

87. Belzer FO, Ashby BS, Huang JS, Dunphy JE: Etiology of rising perfusion pressure in isolated organ perfusion. Ann Surg 1968; 168:382-391.

88. Belzer FO, Ashby BS, Dunphy JE: 24-hour and 72-hour preservation of canine kidneys. Lancet 1967; 2:536-539.

89. Belzer FO, Ashby BS, Gulyassy PF, Powell M: Successful 17-hour preservation and transplantation of human-cadaver kidney. N Engl J Med 1968; 278:608-610.

90. Martin DC, Smith G, Fareed DO: Experimental renal preservation. J Urol 1970; 103:681-685.

91. Nakamoto M, Shapiro JI, Mills SD, Schrier RW, Chan L: Improvement of renal preservation by verapamil with 24-hour cold perfusion in the isolated rat kidney. Transplantation 1988; 45:313-315.

92. Sacks SA, Petritsch PH, Kaufman JJ: Canine kidney preservation using a new perfusate. Lancet 1973; 1:1024-1028.

93. Johnson RWG, Anderson M, Flear CTG, Murray SGH, Taylor RMR, Swinney J: Evaluation of a new perfusion solution for kidney preservation. Transplantation 1972; 13:270-275.

94. Trunkey D, Degenhardt T, Chartrand C, Pryor JP, Belzer FO: Preservation of canine hearts. Cryobiology 1970; 6:515-521.

95. Proctor E, Parker R: Preservation of isolated heart for 72 hours. Br Med J 1968; 4:296-298.

96. Feemster JA, Lillehei RC: Hypothermic-hyperbaric pulsatile perfusion for preservation of the canine heart. Transplant Proc 1969; 1:138-146.

97. Woods JE: Successful three- to seven-day preservation of canine kidneys. Arch Surg 1971; 102:614-616.

98. Van Der Wijk J, Slooff MJH, Rijkmans BG, Kootstra G: Successful 96- and 144-hour experimental kidney preservation: a combination of standard machine preservation and newly developed normothermic ex vivo perfusion. Cryobiology 1980; 17:473-477.

99. Van Der Wijk J, Voordes C, Rijkmans BG, Kootstra G: Light microscopy findings in intermediate term kidney preservation. In: Pegg DE, Jacobsen IA, Halasz NA, eds. Organ Preservation: Basic and Applied Aspects. Boston: MTP Press, 1982:239-243.

100. Bartosek I, Guaitani A, Miller LL: Isolated Liver Perfusion and its Applications. 1st ed. New York: Raven Press, 1973: 87-94.

101. Ritchie HD, Hardcastle JD: Liver. In: Ritchie HD, Hardcastle JD, eds. Isolated Organ Perfusion. London: University Park Press, 1973:71-134.

102. Lambotte L: Liver preservation. In: Toledo-Pereyra LH, ed. Basic Concepts of Organ Procurement, Perfusion, and Preservation. New York: Academic Press, 1982:225-257.

103. Fair JH, Rizzuti RP, Cunningham PR, Thomas FT: Successful hepatic preservation using pulsatile perfusion and allopurinol. Curr Surg 1988; 45:192-194.

104. Pienaar BH, Lindell SL, Van Gulik T, Southard JH, Belzer FO: Seventy-two hour preservation of the canine liver by machine perfusion. Transplantation 1990; 49:258-260.

105. Ritchie HD, Hardcastle JD: Duodenum and pancreas. In: Ritchie HD, Hardcastle JD, eds. Isolated Organ Perfusion. London: University Park Press, 1973:171-208.

106. Martin DR, Scott DF, Downes GL, Belzer FO: Primary cause of unsuccessful liver and heart preservation: cold sensitivity of the ATPase system. Ann Surg 1972; 175:111-117.

107. Kolobow T, Stool EW, Weathersby PK, Pierce J, Hayano F, Suaudeau J: Superior blood compatibility of silicone rubber free of silica filler in the membrane lung. Trans Am Soc Artif Int Organs 1974; 20:269-271.

108. Suaudeau J, Kolobow T: Fresh platelet-rich plasma from a flow-through centrifuge for lamb heart perfusion at 13-degree centigrade. J Thorac Cardiovasc Surg 1976; 72:769-777.

109. Suaudeau J, Kolobow T: Isolated sheep heart hypothermic perfusion with fresh blood: successful preservation for 24-72 hours with continuous strong ventricular activity. Cryobiology 1977; 14:337-348.

110. Guerraty A, Alivizatos P, Warner M, Hess M, Allen L, Lower RR: Successful orthotopic canine heart transplantation after 24 hours of in vitro preservation. J Thorac Cardiovasc Surg 1981; 82:531-537.

111. Choong YS, Gavin JB, Buckman J: Long-term preservation of explanted hearts perfused with L-aspartate-enriched cardioplegic solution. J Thorac Cardiovasc Surg 1992; 103:210-218.

112. Stein DG, Permut LC, Drinkwater DCJr, et al: Complete functional recovery after 24-hour heart preservation with University of Wisconsin solution and modified reperfusion. Circulation 1991; 84 (Suppl. III):316-323.

113. Nutt MP, Fields BL, Belzer FO, Southard JH: Comparison of continuous perfusion and simple cold storage for rabbit heart preservation. Transplant Proc 1991; 23:2445-2446.

114. Burt JM, Copeland JG: Myocardial function after preservation for 24 hours. J Thorac Cardiovasc Surg 1986; 92:238-246.

115. Petsikas D, Mohamed F, Ricci M, Symes J, Guerraty A: Adenosine enhances left ventricular flow during 24-hour hypothermic perfusion of isolated cardiac allografts. J Heart Transplant 1990; 9:543-547.

116. Petsikas D, Ricci MA, Baffour R, de-Varennes B, Symes J, Guerraty A: Enhanced 24-hour in vitro heart preservation with adenosine and adenosine monophosphate. J Heart Transplant 1990; 9:114-118.

117. Wicomb WN, Novitzky D, Cooper DKC, Rose AG: Forty-eight hours hypothermic perfusion storage of pig and baboon hearts. J Surg Res 1986; 40:276-284.

118. Jirsch DW, Fisk RL, Couves CM: Ex vivo evaluation of stored lungs. Ann Thorac Surg 1970; 10:163-168.

119. Haverich A, Scott W, Jamieson SW: Twenty years of lung preservation-a review. Heart Transplant 1985; 4:234-240.

120. Locke TJ, Hooper TL, Flecknell PA, McGregor CGA: Preservation of the lung: comparison of topical cooling and cold crystalloid pulmonary perfusion. J Thorac Cardiovasc Surg 1988; 96:789-795.

121. Modry DL, Jirsch DW, Boehme G, Overton T, Fisk RL, Couves CM: Hypothermic perfusion preservation of the isolated dog lung. Ann Thorac Surg 1973; 16:583-597.

122. Veith FJ, Hagstrom JWC, Nehlsen SL, Karl RC, Deysine M: Functional, hemodynamic, and anatomic changes in isolated perfused dog lungs: the importance of perfusate characteristics. Ann Surg 1967; 165:267-278.

123. Otto TJ, Trenkner M, Stopczyk A, Gawdzinski M, Chelstowska B: Perfusion and ventilation of isolated canine lungs. Thorax 1968; 23:645-651.

124. Taft PM, Collins GM, Grotke GT, Halasz NA: Warm ischemic injury of the lung. J Thorac Cardiovasc Surg 1976; 72:784-787.

125. Adachi H, Ueda K, Koyama I, et al: Donor core cooling for multiple organ retrieval: new application of portable cardiopulmonary bypass for transplantation. Transplant Proc 1989; 21:1200-1202.

126. Starzl TE, Marchioro TL, Von Kaulla KN, Hermann G, Brittain RS, Waddell WR: Homotransplantation of the liver in humans. SGO 1963; 117:659-676.

127. Williams GM, Cameron DE, Fraser CD, et al: Cardiopulmonary bypass with profound hypothermia: an optional preservation method for multi-organ procurement. Transplant Proc 1989; 21:1199-1199.

128. Baumgartner WA, Williams GM, Fraser CDJr, et al: Cardiopulmonary bypass with profound hypothermia. Transplantation 1989; 47:123-127.

129. MacLean LD, Dossetor JB, Gault MH, Oliver JA, Inglis FG, MacKinnon KJ: Renal homotransplantation using cadaver donors. Arch Surg 1965; 91:288-306.

130. Baumgartner WA: Myocardial and pulmonary protection: long-distance transport. Prog Cardiovasc Dis 1990; 33:85-96.

131. Kontos GJJr, Adachi H, Borkon AM, et al: Successful four-hour heart-lung preservation with core-cooling on cardiopulmonary bypass: A simplified model that assesses preservation. J Heart Transplant 1987; 6:106-111.

132. Southard JH, Belzer FO: Kidney preservation by perfusion. In: Cerilli GJ, ed. Organ transplantation and replacement. Philadelphia: J.B. Lippincott Co., 1988:296-311.

133. Belzer FO, Downes GL: Kidney. In: Karow AMJr, Abouna GJM, Humphries ALJr, eds. Organ preservation for transplantation. Boston: Little, Brown & Co., 1974:298-311.

134. Manciet LH, Larson DF, Copeland JG: Low-pressure perfusion results in effective microvascular perfusion of isolated rabbit hearts during hypothermic preservation for twenty-four hours. J Heart Lung Transplant 1991; 10:710-716.

135. Guerraty AJ: Prolonged preservation of the isolated canine heart. Heart Transplant 1981; 1:9-11.

136. Toledo-Pereyra LH: Organ preservation: II. liver, heart, lung, and small intestine. J Surg Res 1981; 30:181-190.

137. Avramovici A: Les Transplantations du rein. Lyon Chir 1924; 21:734-753.

138. Parkinson D, Woodworth HC: Observations on vessel and organ transplants. Exp Med Surg 1947; 5:49-61.

139. Oudot J: Transplantation renale. Presse Med 1948; 56:319-320.

140. Owens JC, Prevedel AE, Swan H: Prolonged experimental occlusion of thoracic aorta during hypothermia. Arch Surg 1955; 70:95-97.

141. Bigelow WG, Lindsay WK, Greenwood WF: Hypothermia. Ann Surg 1950; 132:849-866.

142. Fuhrman FA, Field JII: The reversibility of the inhibition of rat brain and kidney metabolism by cold. Am J Physiol 1943; 139:193-196.

143. Archibald J, Cawley AJ: Some observations on transplantation of the canine kidney. Am J Vet Res 1956; 17:376-379.

144. Schloerb PR, Waldorf RD, Welsh JS: The protective effect of kidney hypothermia on total renal ischemia. SGO 1959; 109:561-565.

145. Kiser JC, Farley HH, Mueller GF, Strobel CJ, Hitchcock CR: Successful renal autografts in the dog after seven hour selective kidney refrigeration. Surg Forum 1960; 11:26-28.

146. Kiser JC, Telander RL, Peterson TA, Coe JI, Hitchcock CR: Canine renal autografts. Arch Surg 1961; 83:502-511.

147. Dempster WJ, Kountz SL, Jovanovic M: Simple kidney-storage technique. Br Med J 1964; 1:407-410.

148. Calne RY, Pegg DE, Pryse-Davies J, Brown FL: Renal preservation by ice-cooling. Br Med J 1963; 2:651-655.

149. Ladaga LG, Nabseth DC, Besznyak I, Hendry WF, McLeod G, Deterling RA: Preservation of canine kidneys by hypothermia and hyperbaric oxygen: long-term survival of autografts following 24-hour storage. Ann Surg 1966; 163:553-558.

150. Manax WG, Lillehei RC: Preservation and storage of mammalian organs. In: Rapaport FT, Dausset J, eds. Human Transplantation. New York: Grune & Stratton, 1968:675-691.

151. Manax WG, Bloch JH, Longerbeam JK, Lillehei RC: Successful 24 hour in vitro preservation of canine kidneys by the combined use of hyperbaric oxygenation and hypothermia. Surgery 1964; 56:275-282.

152. Manax WG, Bloch JH, Eyal Z, Lyons GW, Lillehei RC: Hypothermia and hyperbaria: Simple method for whole organ preservation. JAMA 1965; 192:755-759.

153. Cleveland RJ, Lee HM, Prout GR, Hume DM: Preservation of the cadaver kidney for renal homotransplantation in man. SGO 1964; 119:991-996.

154. Collins GM, Bravo-Shugarman M, Terasaki PI: Kidney preservation for transportation: Initial perfusion and 30 hours' ice storage. Lancet 1969; 2:1219-1222.

155. Schirmer HKA, Walton KN: The effect of hypothermia upon respiration and anaerobic glycolysis of dog kidney. Invest Urol 1964; 1:604-609.

156. Karow AMJr, Webb WR: Cardiac storage with glycerol at zero centigrade. Arch Surg 1961; 83:719-720.

157. Barsamian EM, Win MS, Cady B, Brown H, Collins SC: Preservation of the heart in vitro. In: Brest AN, ed. Heart Substitutes: Mechanical and Transplant. Springfield, Ill: Charles C Thomas, 1966:263-282.

158. Webb WR, Sugg WL, Ecker RR: Heart preservation and transplantation. Am J

Cardiol 1968; 22:820-825.

159. Childs JW, Lower RR: Preservation of the heart. Prog Cardiovasc Dis 1969; 12:149-163.

160. Blumenstock DA, Lempert N, Morgado F: Preservation of the canine lung in vitro for 24 hours with the use of hypothermia and hyperbaric oxygen. J Thorac Cardiovasc Surg 1965; 50:769-774.

161. Toledo-Pereyra LH, Condie RM, Hau T, Simmons RL, Najarian JS: Three-day hypothermic storage of canine lungs. Surg Forum 1977; 28:194-195.

162. Mancini MC, Griffith BP, Borovetz HS, Hardesty RL: Static lung preservation. Curr Surg 1985; 42:23-25.

163. Keeler R, Swinney J, Taylor RMR, Uldell PR: The problem of renal preservation. Br J Urol 1966; 38:653-656.

164. Collins GM: Flush preservation. In: Pegg DE, Jacobsen IA, Halasz NA, eds. Organ preservation: Basic and applied aspects. Boston: MTP Press, 1982:167-177.

165. Collins GM, Halasz NA: Forty-eight hour ice storage of kidneys: Importance of cation content. Surgery 1976; 79:432-435.

166. Collins GM, Green RD, Halasz NA: Importance of anion content and osmolarity in flush solutions for 48 to 72 hour hypothermic kidney storage. Cryobiology 1979; 16:217-220.

167. Thomas FT, Szentpetery SS, Mammana RE, Wolfgang TC, Lower RR: Long-distance transportation of human hearts for transplantation. Ann Thorac Surg 1978; 26:344-350.

168. Toledo-Pereyra LH, Chee M, Condie RM, Najarian JS, Lillehei RC: Forty-eight hours hypothermic storage of whole canine pancreas allografts. Improved preservation with a colloid hyperosmolar solution. Cryobiology 1979; 16:221-228.

169. Squifflet JP, Pirson Y, Gianello P, Van Cangh P, Alexandre GPJ: Safe preservation of human renal cadaver transplants by Euro-Collins solution up to 50 hours. Transplant Proc 1981; 13:693-696.

170. Vaughn WK, Mendez-Picon G, Humphries AL, Spees EK: Method of preservation is not a determinant of graft outcome in kidneys transplanted by Southeastern Organ Procurement Foundation institutions. Transplanta-

tion 1981; 32:490-494.

171. Wahlberg JA, Love R, Landegaard L, Southard JH, Belzer FO: 72-hour preservation of the canine pancreas. Transplantation 1987; 43:5-8.

172. Levy MN: Oxygen consumption and blood flow in the hypothermic, perfused kidney. Am J Physiol 1959; 197:1111-1114.

173. Schueler S, Warnecke H, Hetzer R, Loitz F, Topalidis T, Borst HG: The limits of cold ischemia for preservation of the lung. J Heart Transplant 1984; 4:70-75.

174. Hachida M, Morton DL: A new solution (UCLA formula) for lung preservation. J Thorac Cardiovasc Surg 1989; 97:513-520.

175. Hooper TL, Locke TJ, Fetherston G, Flecknell PA, McGregor CGA: Comparison of cold flush perfusion with modified blood versus modified Euro-Collins solution for lung preservation. J Heart Transplant 1990; 9:429-434.

176. Connaughton PJ, Bahuth JJ, Lewis FJ: Lung ischemia up to six hours; influence of local cooling in situ on subsequent pulmonary function. Dis Chest 1962; 41:404-408.

177. Bonser RS, Fischel R, Fragomeni L, et al: Successful human double-lung transplantation after five and one-half hours of preservation. J Thorac Cardiovasc Surg 1989; 98:942-944.

178. Hachida M, Morton DL: Lung function after prolonged lung preservation. J Thorac Cardiovasc Surg 1989; 97:911-919.

179. Hall TS, Borkon AM, Gurtner GC, et al: Improved static lung preservation with corticosteroids and hypothermia. J Heart Transplant 1988; 7:348-352.

180. Keshavjee SH, Yamazaki F, Yokomise H, et al: The role of dextran 40 and potassium in extended hypothermic lung preservation for transplantation. J Thorac Cardiovasc Surg 1992; 103:314-325.

181. Lambert CJ, Egan TM, Detterbeck FC, Keagy BA, Wilcox BR: Enhanced pulmonary function using dimethylthiourea for twelve-hour lung preservation. Ann Thorac Surg 1991; 51:924-930.

182. Jeevanandam V, Auteri JS, Sanchez JA, et al: Improved heart preservation with University of Wisconsin solution: experimental and preliminary human experience. Circulation 1991;

84 (Suppl. III):324-328.

183. Bonser RS, Rotenberg D, Fragomeni LS, Fischel R, Jamieson SW, Kaye MP: Pharmacologic manipulation of elevated pulmonary vascular resistance following 12-hour lung preservation. Transplant Proc 1990; 22:555-556.

184. Fujimura S, Handa M, Kondo T, Ichinose T, Shiraishi Y, Nakada T: Successful 48-hour simple hypothermic preservation of canine lung transplants. Transplant Proc 1987; 19:1334-1336.

185. Miyoshi S, Shimokawa S, Schreinemakers H, et al: Comparison of the University of Wisconsin preservation solution and other crystalloid perfusates in a 30-hour rabbit lung preservation model. J Thorac Cardiovasc Surg 1992; 103:27-32.

186. Veith FJ, Crane R, Torres M, et al: Effective preservation and transportation of lung transplants. J Thorac Cardiovasc Surg 1976; 72:97-105.

187. Crane R, Torres M, Hagstrom JWC, Koerner SK, Veith FJ: Twenty-four-hour preservation and transplantation of the lung without functional impairment. Surg Forum 1975; 26:111-113.

188. Breda MA, Hall TS, Stuart RS, et al: Twenty-four hour lung preservation by hypothermia and leukocyte depletion. Heart Transplant 1985; 4:325-329.

189. Yacoub MH, Khaghani A, Banner N, Tajkarimi S, Fitzgerald M: Distant organ procurement for heart and lung transplantation. Transplant Proc 1989; 21:2548-2550.

190. Jeevanandam V, Barr ML, Auteri JS et al: University of Wisconsin solution versus crystalloid cardioplegia for human donor heart preservation. J Thorac Cardiovasc Surg 1992; 103:194-199.

191. Stein DG, Drinkwater DCJr, Laks H et al: Cardiac preservation in patients undergoing transplantation. A clinical trial comparing University of Wisconsin solution and Stanford solution. J Thorac Cardiovasc Surg 1991; 102:657-665.

192. Kawahara K, Ikari H, Hisano H et al: Twenty-four-hour canine lung preservation using UW solution. Transplantation 1991; 51:584-587.

193. Semik M, Moller F, Lange V, Bernhard A, Toomes H: Comparison of Euro-Collins and UW-1 solutions for lung preservation using the parabiotic rat perfusion model. Transplant Proc 1990; 22:2235-2236.

194. Okouchi Y, Shimizu K, Yamaguchi A, Kamada N: Effectiveness of modified University of Wisconsin solution for heart preservation as assessed in heterotopic rat heart transplant model. J Thorac Cardiovasc Surg 1990; 99:1104-1108.

195. Wang G, Reader J, Hynd J, Pepper J: Improved heart and lung preservation in a rat model. Transpl Int 1990; 3:206-211.

196. Pegg DE: The principles of organ storage procedures. In: Pegg DE, Jacobsen IA, Halasz NA, eds. Organ Preservation: Basic and Applied Aspects. Boston: MTP Press, 1982:55-66.

197. Jacobsen IA, Kemp E, Buhl MR: An adverse effect of rapid cooling in kidney preservation. Transplantation 1979; 27:135-136.

198. Walker WF, Macdonald JS, Pickard C: Hepatic vein sphincter mechanism in the dog. Brit J surg 1960; 48:218-220.

199. Whittembury G, Proverbio F: Two models of Na extrusion in cells from guinea pig kidney cortex slices. Pflugers Arch 1970; 316:1-25.

200. Ackermann JRW, Barnard CN: Successful storage of kidneys. Br J Surg 1966; 53:525-532.

201. Lillehei RC, Manax WG, Bloch JH, Eyal Z, Hidalgo F, Longerbeam JK: In vitro preservation of whole organs by hypothermia and hyperbaric oxygenation. Cryobiology 1964; 1:181-193.

202. Lokkegaard H: Kidney preservation with hypothermia and hyperbaric oxygen. Acta Med Scand 1970; 187:195-202.

203. Hitchcock CR, Haglin JJ, Telander RL, Shapiro FL, Simso LA: Hyperbaric oxygenation in surgery. Arch Surg 1965; 91:307-313.

204. Taylor AC: The physical state transition in the freezing of living cells. Ann NY Acad Sci 1960; 85:595-609.

205. Norman JN, Smith G, Douglas TA: The effect of oxygen at elevated atmospheric pressure and hypothermia on tissue metabolism. SGO 1966; 122:778-784.

206. Lillehei RC: Preservation of organs. In: Mitchison NA, Greep JM, Verschure JCMH, eds. Organ Transplantation Today. Balti-

more: The Williams & Wilkins Co., 1969:109-113.

207. Smith AU: Studies on golden hamsters during cooling to and rewarming from body temperatures below 0 C. II. Observations during and after resuscitation. Proc R Soc Lond (Biol) 1956; 145B:407-426.

208. Ding ZK, Sumrani N, Hong JH: Prolonged simple cryothermic immersion storage of rat heart isografts: a preliminary study. J Invest Surg 1991; 4:171-174.

209. Wang TC, Connery CP, Batty PR, Hicks GL, DeWeere JA Jr, Layne JR: Freezing preservation of adult mammalian heart at high subzero temperatures. Cryobiology 1991; 28:171-176.

210. Mundth ED, DeFalco AJ, Jacobson YG: Functional survival of kidneys subjected to extracorporeal freezing and reimplantation. Cryobiology 1965; 2:62-67.

211. Lehr HB: Progress in long-term organ freezing. Transplant Proc 1971; 3:1565-1568.

212. Guttman FM, Lizin J, Robitaille P, Blanchard H, Turgeon-Knaack C: Survival of canine kidneys after treatment with dimethyl-sulfoxide, freezing at -80 C, and thawing by microwave illumination. Cryobiology 1977; 14:559-567.

213. Dietzman RH, Rebelo AE, Graham EF, Grabo BG, Lillehei RC: Long-term functional success following freezing of canine kidneys. Surgery 1973; 74:181-189.

214. Karow AM Jr: Problems of organ cryopreservation. In: Karow AM Jr, Pegg DE, eds. Organ Preservation for Transplantation. 2nd ed. New York: Marcel, Dekker, Inc., 1981:517-552.

215. Pegg DE, Green CJ, Walter CA: Attempted canine renal cryopreservation using dimethyl sulphoxide helium perfusion and microwave thawing. Cryobiology 1978; 15:618-626. (Abstract)

216. Mehl PM: Experimental dissection of devitrification in aqueous solutions of 1,3-butanediol. Cryobiology 1990; 27:378-400.

217. Fahy GM, Saur J, Williams RJ: Physical problems with the vitrification of large biological systems. Cryobiology 1990; 27:492-510.

218. Ruggera PS, Fahy GM: Rapid and uniform electromagnetic heating of aqueous cryoprotectant solutions from cryogenic temperatures. Cryobiology 1990; 27:465-478.

219. Pegg DE: Principles of tissue preservation. In: Morris PJ, Tilney NL, eds. Progress in Transplantation. London: Churchill Livingstone, 1985:69-105.

220. Baitz T, Hallenbeck GA, Shorter RG, Scott GW, Owen CA, Hunt JC: Preservation of kidneys for transplantation. Arch Surg 1965; 91:276-287.

221. Fahy GM, Hirsch A: Prospects for organ preservation by vitrification. In: Pegg DE, Jacobsen IA, Halasz NA, eds. Organ preservation: Basic and Applied Aspects. Boston: MTP Press, 1982:399-404.

222. Pegg DE, Jacobsen IA and Halasz NA: Organ Preservation. 1st ed. Boston: MTP Press Ltd., 1982.405-421.

223. Marcus E, Wong SNT, Luisada AA: Homologous heart grafts. Arch Surg 1953; 66:179-191.

224. Lavender AR, Berndt AA, Stupka JJ: Extracorporeal renal transplantation. Trans Am Soc Artif Int Organs 1966; 12:246-253.

225. Gilsdorf RB, Clark SD, Leonard AS: Extracorporeal recipient shunt homograft kidney perfusion, a model for organ resuscitation and function evaluation. Trans Am Soc Artif Int Organs 1965; 11:219-224.

226. Belin RP, Gilsdorf RB, Clark SD, Leonard AS: Recipient shunt ex vivo hypothermic perfusion model for organ preservation and dialysis. Trans Am Soc Artif Int Organs 1966; 12:254-258.

227. Angell WW, Dong E, Shumway NE: Four-day storage of the canine cadaver heart. Rev Surg 1968; 25:369-370.

228. Brull L, Louis-Bar D: Toxicity of artificially circulated heparinized blood on the kidney. Arch Int Physiol Biochim 1957; 65:470-476.

229. Knowlton FP, Starling EH: The influence of variations in temperature and blood-pressure on the performance of the isolated mammalian heart. J Physiol (London) 1912; 44:206-219.

230. Bainbridge FA, Evans CL: The heart, lung, kidney preparation. J Physiol (London) 1914; 48:278-286.

231. Canny AJ, Verney EB, Winton FR: The double heart-lung-kidney preparation. J Physiol (London) 1930; 68:333-347.

232. Sen PK, Shah CB, Satoskar RS: Studies on isolated heart-lung preparations in the hypothermic animal. J Intern Coll Surg 1956; 26:32-37.

233. Webb WR, Howard HS: Cardiopulmonary transplantation. Surg Forum 1957; 8:313-317.

234. Robicsek F, Sanger PW, Taylor FH: Simple method of keeping the heart "alive" and functioning outside of the body for prolonged periods. Surgery 1963; 53:525-530.

235. Robicsek F, Pruitt JR, Sanger PW, Daugherty HK, Moore M, Bagby E: The maintenance of function of the donor heart in the extracorporeal stage and during transplantation. Ann Thorac Surg 1968; 6:330-342.

236. Whiffen JD, Boake WC, Gott VL: Normothermic orthotopic canine heart homotransplantation. J Surg Res 1967; 7:421-426.

237. Wuerflein RD, Shumway NE: Resuscitation and function of the cadaver heart. Circulation 1967; 35 (Suppl.I):92-95.

238. Yamada T, Bosher LH, Richardson GM: Observations on the autoperfusing heart-lung preparation. Trans Am Soc Artif Int Organs 1965; 11:192-196.

239. Wicomb WN, Cooper DKC: Donor heart storage. In: Cooper DKC, Lanza RP, eds. Heart Transplantation. Boston: MTP Press Ltd., 1984:51-76.

240. Robicsek F, Tam W, Daugherty HK, Robicsek LK: The stabilized autoperfusion heart-lung preparation as a vehicle for extracorporeal preservation. Transplant Proc 1969; 1:834-839.

241. Tam W, Robicsek F, Daugherty HK, Mullen DC: Autoperfusing heart-lung preparation: prolonged survival by extracorporeal symbiosis. Transplant Proc 1971; 3:640-642.

242. Hutter JA, Higenbottam T, Wallwork J: Cardiopulmonary preservation. J Heart Transplant 1988; 7:312-313.

243. Morimoto T, Golding LR, Stewart RW, et al: A simple method for extended heart-lung preservation by autoperfusion. Trans Am Soc Artif Int Organs 1984; 30:320-324.

244. Robicsek F, Masters TN, Duncan GD, Denyer MH, Rise HE, Etchison M: An autoperfused heart-lung-preparation: metabolism and function. Heart Transplant 1985; 4:334-338.

245. Riveron FA, Ross JH, Schwartz KA, et al: Energy expenditure of autoperfusing heart-lung preparation. Circulation 1988; 78 (Suppl. III):103-109.

246. Kontos GJ, Borkon AM, Baumgartner WA et al: Improved myocardial and pulmonary preservation by metabolic substrate enhancement in the autoperfused working heart-lung preparation. J Heart Transplant 1988; 7:140-144.

247. Naka Y, Hirose H, Matsuda H, et al: Prevention of pulmonary edema in autoperfusing heart-lung preparation by FUT-175 and leukocyte depletion. Transplant Proc 1989; 21:1353-1356.

248. Kontos GJ, Borkon AM, Adachi H, et al: Successful extended cardiopulmonary preservation in the autoperfused working heart-lung preparation. Surgery 1987; 102:269-276.

249. Adachi H, Fraser CD, Kontos GJ, et al: Autoperfused working heart-lung preparation versus hypothermic cardiopulmonary preservation for transplantation. J Heart Transplant 1987; 6:253-260.

250. Cooper DKC: A simple method of resuscitation and short-term preservation of the canine cadaver heart. J Thorac Cardiovasc Surg 1975; 70:896-908.

251. Ladowski JS, Kapelanski DP, Teodori MF, Stevenson WC, Hardesty RL, Griffith BP: Use of autoperfusion for distant procurement of heart-lung allografts. Heart Transplant 1985; 4:330-333.

252. Griffith BP, Hardesty RL, Trento A, et al: Heart-lung transplantation: Lessons learned and future hopes. Ann Thorac Surg 1987; 43:6-16.

253. Dupree EL, Milles M, Clark R, Sell KW: Xenogeneic storage of primate hearts. Transplant Proc 1969; 1:840-851.

254. Stewart RW, Morimoto T, Golding LR, Harasaki H, Olsen E, Nose Y: Canine heart-lung autoperfusion. Trans Am Soc Artif Int Organs 1985; 31:206-210.

255. Chien S, Diana JN, Todd EP, O'Connor WN, Marion T, Smith K: New autoperfusion preparation for long-term organ preservation. Circulation 1988; 78 (Suppl. III):58-65.

256. Robicsek F: Cardiopulmonary preservation. J Heart Transplant 1988; 7:313-313.

257. Kresh JY, Brockman SK: Autoperfusing ec-

tothermic heart-lung preservation system. J Invest Surg 1989; 2:281-291.

258. Chien S, Todd EP, Diana JN, O'Connor WN: A simple technique for multiorgan preservation. J Thorac Cardiovasc Surg 1988; 95:55-61.

259. Chien S, Diana JN, Oeltgen PR, Todd EP, O'Connor WN: Eighteen to 37 hours' preservation of major organs using a new autoperfusion multiorgan preparation. Ann Thorac Surg 1989; 47:860-867.

260. Chien S, Diana JN, Oeltgen PR, Salley R: Functional studies of the heart during a 24-hour preservation using a new autoperfusion preparation. J Heart Lung Transplant 1991; 10:401-408.

261. Chien S, Oeltgen PR, Diana JN, Shi X, Nilekani SP, Salley R: Two-day preservation of major organs with autoperfusion multiorgan preparation and hibernation induction trigger. J Thorac Cardiovasc Surg 1991; 102:224-234.

262. Chien S, Oeltgen PR, Su TP, Diana JN, Salley R: Delta opiold DADLE extended tissue survival time in multiorgan block preservation. J Thorac Cardiovasc Surg 1992; (In Press)

263. Minten J, Segel LD, Van-Belle H, Wynants J, Flameng W: Differences in high-energy phosphate catabolism between the rat and the dog in a heart preservation model. J Heart Lung Transplant 1991; 10:71-78.

264. Havel M, Owen AN, Simon P: Basic principles of cardioplegic management in donor heart preservation. Clin Ther 1991; 13:289-303.

265. Kaye MP: The registry of the International Society for Heart Transplantation: fourth official report-1987. J Heart Transplant 1987; 6:63-67.

266. Lurie KG, Billingham ME, Masek MA, et al:

Ultrastructural and functional studies on prolonged myocardial preservation in an experimental heart transplant model. J Thorac Cardiovasc Surg 1982; 84:122-129.

267. Takahashi A, Braimbridge MV, Hearse DJ, Chambers DJ: Long-term preservation of the mammalian myocardium. Effect of storage medium and temperature on the vulnerability to tissue injury. J Thorac Cardiovasc Surg 1991; 102:235-245.

268. Doring V, Schaper J, Stubbe HM: Postischemic recovery of the lung-biochemical and morphological studies of long-term preserved lungs. Transplant Proc 1991; 23:2347-2349.

269. Takahashi A, Hearse DJ, Braimbridge MV, Chambers DJ: Harvesting hearts for long-term preservation. J Thorac Cardiovasc Surg 1990; 100:371-378.

270. Chambers DJ, Takahashi A, Hearse DJ: Long-term preservation of the heart: the effect of infusion pressure during continuous hypothermic cardioplegia. J Heart Lung Transplant 1992; 11:665-675.

271. Mollhoff T, Sukehiro S, Van Aken H, Flameng W: Long-term preservation of baboon hearts: Effects of hypothermic ischemic and cardioplegic arrest on high energy phosphate content. Circulation 1990; 82 (Suppl. IV):264-268.

272. Milliken JC, Billingsley AM, Laks H: Modified reperfusate after long-term preservation of the heart. Ann Thorac Surg 1989; 47:725-728.

273. McAnulty JF, Ploeg RJ, Southard JH, Belzer FO: Successful five-day perfusion preservation of the canine kidney. Transplantation 1989; 47:37-41.

274. Ross BD: Future prospects in organ preservation. In: Pegg DE, Jacobsen IA, Halasz NA, eds. Organ preservation: Basic and Applied Aspects. Boston: MTP Press, 1982:103-108.

CHAPTER 3

Technique for Harvesting and Preserving a Multiorgan Block Preparation

Multiorgan block harvesting removes six organs from the chest and abdomen. It is preferable for two surgical teams to be involved in the procedure. One team performs the operation in the abdomen, while another removes the organs from the chest. The technique described herein is for a one-team operation only, although the procedure is similar when two teams participate.

PREOPERATIVE PREPARATION

Before the surgery, oral antibiotics are administered to sterilize the gastrointestinal tract. We usually give each animal neomycin (2 gm per day) for three days before surgery. Five hours before surgery, the animal should be fasted. The stomach enlarges substantially after eating, making it more difficult to dissect and increasing the chance for leakage of contents during removal.

Anesthesia

Any general anesthesia is satisfactory for the surgery. We usually use sodium pentobarbital (30 mg/kg, iv). It is usually not necessary to supplement with additional doses, but 5-10 mg/kg can be administered as required to maintain a surgical plane of anesthesia. An endotracheal tube is inserted, and artificial ventilation is maintained during the surgery with a gas mixture of 50% oxygen, 3% carbon dioxide and 47% nitrogen. PEEP is not needed during the operation.

Position and Preparation

The animal is placed in a supine position with all four legs restrained. We prefer to place one catheter in the femoral artery for arterial pressure monitoring and another catheter in the femoral vein for fluid infusion and blood sampling during the operation. The monitoring and transfusion catheters are switched to the splenic artery and vein before the abdominal aorta and inferior vena cava are ligated.

SURGICAL PROCEDURE

INCISION

A midline incision is suitable for both the chest and abdominal procedures. When one team does the surgery, the abdominal surgery is performed first to reduce lung exposure. When lung tissue is exposed to air for a long period of time, it will dry out quickly, resulting in lung damage before the preservation period. If two operating teams are available, the chest and abdominal operations are performed at the same time. Using this two-team approach, the organ block can be removed within an hour. This decreases operative time, reduces tissue damage, and extends organ survival.

ABDOMINAL SURGERY

After the abdomen is opened, a large retractor is used to hold the abdominal wall open. We use a special rectangular retractor with four blades attached to it. (Fig. 1) This retractor can keep the abdomen fully open without much weight on the animal.

The dissection begins from the small intestine. The duodenum with the pancreas attached is identified. Two umbilical tape ties are placed at the lower part of the duodenum, and the intestine is separated between the ties. (Fig. 2) The colon is pulled towards the pelvis, and the dissection to divide the mesentery is carried out towards the left of the abdomen. The retroperitoneum is opened over the left kidney and the abdominal aorta. The superior mesenteric artery and vein are located. (Fig. 3) Careful dissection is employed to expose the superior mesenteric artery and to dissect it over as long a segment as possible. The artery is divided between two clamps, and double 2-0 silk ties are used to ligate both ends. The dissection of the mesentery is carried down until it reaches the sigmoid, where the inferior mesenteric vessels are separated and ligated. (Fig. 4) The sigmoid is detached from the rectum between two umbilical tape ties. Thus, the whole intestinal blood is connected to the body by only a pedicle containing the superior mesenteric vein. The intestines are held high to allow most of the blood to return to the circulation. (Fig. 5) The pedicle is then tied and disconnected, and the intestines are removed from the abdomen.

The omentum is separated between the stomach and the spleen. The splenic artery is ligated, and an 8F catheter is inserted into the splenic artery for arterial pressure measurement and arterial blood sampling. The spleen is held in an elevated position for several seconds to allow most of the blood in the spleen to return to the body. Another 8F catheter is inserted into the portal vein ac-

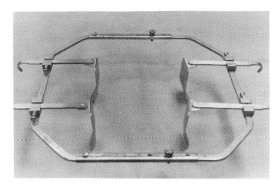

Fig. 1. The rectangular retractor used for abdominal surgery. The four blades are retractable to accommodate different incision sizes.

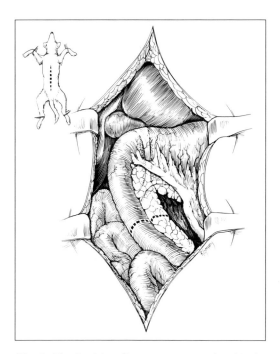

Fig. 2. The incision line to separate the duodenum from the jejunum. The insert shows the abdominal incision line.

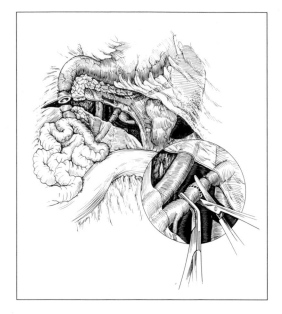

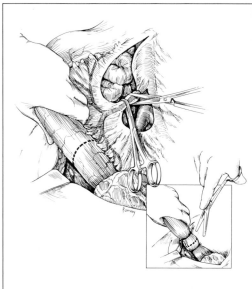

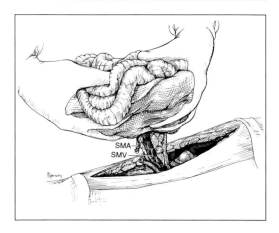

cessed via the splenic vein for portal vein pressure measurement and infusion of fluid. (Fig. 6) The spleen is then removed from the body. The lesser omentum is divided and ligated with the right and left gastric vessels. The right and left crura of the diaphragm are divided, and the gastrophrenic ligament is detached. The stomach is then removed by dividing the esophagus from the stomach below the diaphragm and disconnecting the duodenum from the pylorus. (Fig. 7)

At this time the abdomen is clear for dissection of the organs to be included in the preservation block. The left kidney is dissected free. All the severed tissue on the kidney must be ligated to prevent oozing of blood when the kidney is placed in the bath solution. The ureter is separated from the surrounding tissue but is not cut at this time. The renal artery and vein are dissected free up to the abdominal aorta and the inferior vena cava (IVC). It is not necessary to remove all fat tissue around the kidney and its vessels. (Fig. 8) The adrenal gland may be left attached to the organ block. The right kidney is dissected free using the same technique.

The abdominal aorta and inferior vena cava are then dissected free by dividing and ligating their lumbar branches. The lumbar veins are very thin and fragile. Only one or two vessels may be clamped at one time, and fine ligatures must be used to reduce the

---

Fig. 3. (Top left) The duodenum is separated from the jejunum, and the retroperitoneum is opened to expose the superior mesenteric vessels. The insert shows the separation of the superior mesenteric artery. The mesenteric vein is left attached to allow venous blood to return from the intestine.

Fig. 4. (Middle left) The dissection of the inferior mesenteric vessels and the incision line of the sigmoid. The insert shows the cut line of the sigmoid.

Fig. 5. (Bottom left) After the duodenum and sigmoid are separated and the mesentery is cut. The intestines are held in an elevated position to allow more blood to come back from the intestines. The superior mesenteric vein is then divided and ligated to remove the intestines.

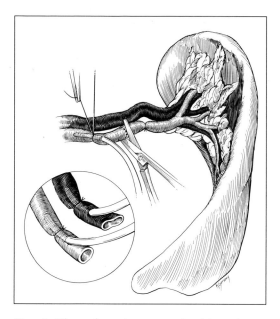

Fig. 6. The spleen is removed with catheters inserted into the splenic artery and vein for pressure measurements, blood sampling, and fluid infusions.

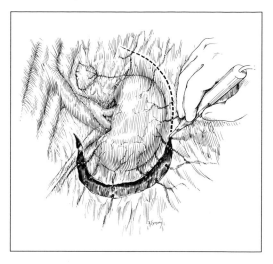

Fig. 8. The dissection of the left kidney is performed by dividing the retroperitoneum. All the blood-supplying vessels should be ligated to prevent later bleeding.

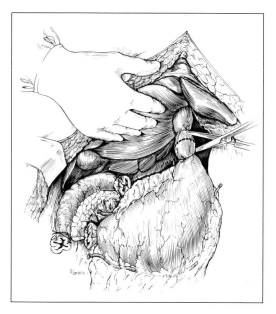

Fig. 7. The diaphragm is separated from the stomach, which is then separated from the esophagus and removed.

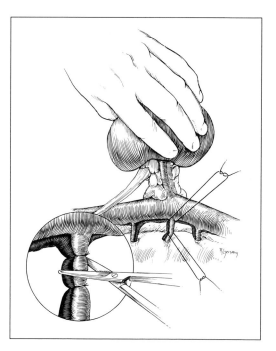

Fig. 9. The dissection of the abdominal aorta and inferior vena cava is accomplished by dividing lumbar vessels. These vessels should be divided and ligated carefully to avoid bleeding.

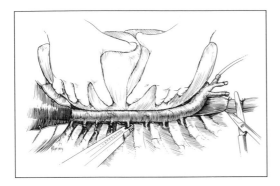

Fig. 10. The dissection of the descending aorta is accomplished by dividing the intercostal arteries. Using LDS powered staplers can speed up the procedure and reduce operative time.

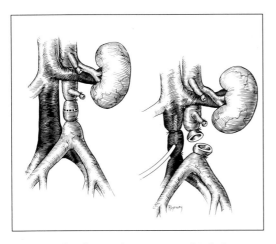

Fig. 11. The descending aorta and inferior vena cava are separated, and a catheter is inserted into the IVC for pressure measurement, fluid infusion and blood sampling.

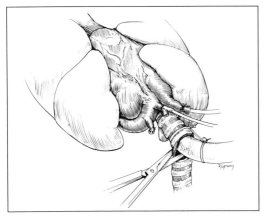

Fig. 12. The trachea is cut and an endotracheal tube is inserted for artificial ventilation.

chance of bleeding. (Fig. 9) The diaphragm covering the abdominal aorta and the inferior vena cava is also detached and carefully ligated. Thus, the duodenum, pancreas, both kidneys and part of the liver are free from attachments to the body.

CHEST OPERATION

The midline abdominal incision is extended to the chest through a median sternotomy. The mediastinal tissue over the pericardium is divided and ligated along with the internal mammary arteries. The thymus is removed because it tends to become necrotic during preservation. A large chest retractor is used to open the incision. The diaphragm is divided and ligated around the liver and the inferior vena cava. After the liver is truncated from its supporting tissue, it tends to move out of position, stretching or kinking the hepatic vein and the inferior vena cava. Support may be needed to maintain correct liver alignment so that circulatory disturbance is reduced to a minimum.

The descending aorta is dissected free from the chest. All the intercostal branches are divided and ligated individually. The dissection of the descending aorta requires displacement of the whole left lung and the heart to the right side, which always creates a circulation disturbance. To speed up the dissection and reduce blood pressure fluctuations, we prefer to use an LDS powered stapler (United States Surgical, Norwalk, CT) for fast cutting of the intercostal arteries. (Fig. 10) The dissection of the descending aorta is carried up to the left subclavian artery, which is also divided and ligated. The esophagus is separated from the body by dividing it at the level of the aortic arch. The esophagus can be left with the organ block and removed later when the organ block is placed in the bath, where the esophagus is exposed on the surface. On the right side, the azygos vein is divided and ligated below its junction with the superior vena cava. The inferior vena cava is dissected free. If blood pressure is still sufficiently elevated at this time, a blood-collecting bag containing CPDA solution is connected to the left subclavian artery and positioned 100 cm above the heart.

The bag is used to collect excess blood when the circulation to the body is disconnected. It is removed before the organs are disconnected from the body. Low blood pressure during the operation is usually the result of blood loss; infusion of fluids should be instituted. We have found that excessive blood transfusion during harvesting tends to augment liver congestion. Crystalloid solutions, such as lactated Ringers' solution, are usually satisfactory for volume replacement. The abdominal aorta is divided and ligated below its renal branches. The hind legs are lifted for several minutes to allow more blood to return to the circulation. The inferior vena cava is then ligated and divided at the same level as the aorta, and an 8F catheter is placed in the IVC for venous blood pressure measurement and blood sampling. (Fig. 11) The right innominate artery is divided and ligated, and an 8F catheter is inserted through it into the left ventricle for left ventricular pressure measurement and dp/dt monitoring. The superior vena cava is divided and ligated. The trachea is transected, and an endotracheal tube is inserted for ventilation. (Fig. 12) The heart, lungs, liver, duodenum, pancreas and both kidneys are disconnected from the body while they are still perfused by the heart and oxygenated by the lungs. Before the organ block is removed from the body, the following procedures are performed:

1. The left and right ureters are cut, and two 5F catheters are placed in the ureters for collecting urine.

2. One 8F catheter is placed in the common bile duct to collect bile. (Fig. 13)

3. One plastic tube 3/8" in diameter is placed in the duodenum to collect pancreatic and duodenal fluids.

Transporting the Organ Block to the Bath Solution

A piece of wet towel is passed through the space between the back of the organ block and the animal's body. This towel is used to cradle the whole organ block when it is removed from the body. (Fig. 14) The whole system as shown in Figure 15 is then transferred from the body and placed in a bath solution. The position of the organ block in the bath solution should be resemble its normal position in a standing animal. That is, the back side of the organ block is on the surface, with the lungs floating on the bath water surface and the heart hanging below. Any remaining bleeding vessels should be ligated at this time, because the original back

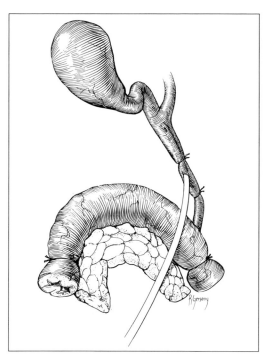

Fig. 13. The common bile duct is cannulated with a 8F catheter for collecting the bile. The tip of the catheter should not be advanced into the gallbladder.

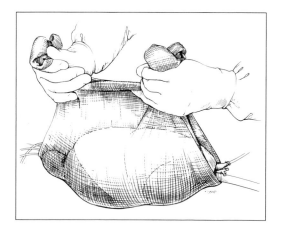

Fig. 14. A large towel is used to cradle the organ block to transport the organ block from the body to bath tank.

side is now on the surface. The esophagus is removed at this time if desired.

When the organ block is placed in the bath solution, the heart and liver tend to sink to the bottom of the bath while the lungs float on the surface. This can cause stretching and/or kinking of the blood vessels, especially the hepatic vein and the inferior vena cava. To correctly align the organs, we use laboratory ringstands for the liver and kidneys. (Fig. 16) The liver and kidneys are placed on the stands, and the solution level is adjusted so

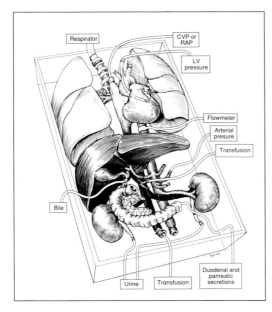

Fig. 15. The finished multiorgan block with all the catheters inserted is shown here. Note that when the organ block is placed in the bath solution, the block should be placed in an upside-down position. That is, the lungs float on the surface of the bath solution and the heart hangs at the bottom.

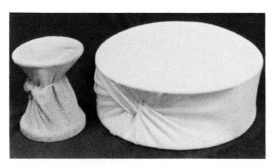

Fig. 16. Laboratory ringstands are used to support the liver and kidneys. The stands are covered by fabrics.

that the organs are well aligned and the blood vessels are straight. (Fig. 17) In this way liver congestion can be reduced or eliminated and proper circulation maintained. No inotropic drugs are necessary. To keep the organ block in a temperature-controlled and sterile condition, we use a special container for the organ block. The container is made of 4 mm plexiglass with two chambers. The inner chamber, which is 14" wide x 12" deep x 10" high, is lined with a sterile plastic bag, and bath solution is placed in this bag. The outer chamber is 4 inches larger than the inner chamber around the periphery. This outer chamber contains a temperature-controlled heating pump and circulating water. (Fig. 18) Before each experiment, only the plastic lining bag must be sterilized. The bath solution contains 10-12 liters of lactated Ringer's solution, 100 mg of heparin sodium, 1,000 mg of neomycin, and 1,000,000 units of penicillin. The pH is adjusted to 7.35-7.45.

SPECIAL MEASURES TO ENSURE ASEPTIC PRESERVATION

The preservation environment provides an excellent medium for bacterial growth, that is, the physiologic solution contains blood and protein, the medium contains living tissues, and the entire block is maintained at a suitable temperature. Bacteria can be introduced into the blood circulation or can grow in the preservation solution and eventually enter the organ block. To reduce the risk of infection, special attention must be paid before, during and after the harvesting procedure:

1. Pretreatment:

Oral antibiotics are administered before the operation as previously described.

2. During harvesting:

a) Skin preparation: good shaving of the skin and sterilization of the chest and abdominal walls are required. Using surface bactericides such as iodine or Betadine soap and alcohol preparation for the skin incisions has proven effective.

b) Drapes and instrumentation: all drapes and instruments are sterilized.

c) Treatment of gastrointestinal tract: when

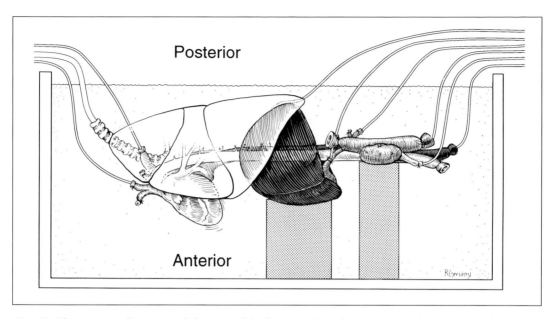

Fig. 17. The correct alignment of the organ block when placed in the bath solution. Special attention is paid to the inferior vena cava between the heart and the liver. This portion is vulnerable to kinks and distortion if the organs are not aligned correctly.

the incision is made in the gastrointestinal tract, disinfectant solution must be used to sterilize the incision to reduce bacterial contamination.

3. *During preservation:*

a) Bath solution and container: the container and bath solution are sterile.

b) Blood and fluids: all blood should be obtained and transfused aseptically.

c) Infusion sets and catheters: all equipment is sterilized and indwelling catheters are changed every 24 hours.

d) Intravenous antibiotics: Appropriate antibiotics should be given intravenously. We usually give ampicillin (50 mg) by intravenous infusion every 12 hours and Flagyl (500 mg in 1000 ml solution) as a continuous drip.

MONITORING AND INTERVENTION DURING PRESERVATION

In this preparation, all the organs are functioning during both harvesting and preservation. This feature provides an opportunity for continuous monitoring of organ function. Monitoring of each organ can be simple or sophisticated, depending on the purpose. If the preservation is for functional studies, more parameters should be moni-

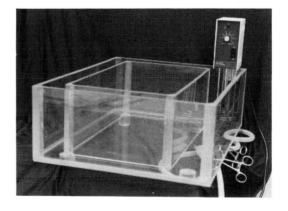

Fig. 18. The plexiglass tank used for the organ block.

tored and, consequently, more manipulation is needed. On the other hand, if transplantation into a donor is the final goal, only basic parameters are needed, and the organs are disturbed less frequently. The following parameters are monitored in most of our experiments:

1. *Heart function:*
a) Aortic pressure
b) Left ventricular pressure
c) Central venous pressure
d) Left ventricular dp/dt

e) Right ventricular pressure
f) Aortic blood flow
g) Pulmonary artery blood flow
h) Left ventricular diameter or dimension

2. Lung mechanical function:

a) Tidal volume
b) Inspiratory pressure
c) Air flow

3. Blood chemistries:

Blood samples are taken before and immediately after the operation and every 4 hours during the preservation time.

a) Routine chemistry: potassium, sodium, chloride, calcium, glucose, lactic acid, pyruvate, osmolarity, protein, albumin and uric acid.

b) Enzymes for organ function: aspartate amino-transferase (AST), alanine amino-transferase (ALT), lactic dehydrogenase (LDH) and its isoenzymes, alkaline phosphatase (ALP), gamma glutamyl transpeptidase (GGT), creatine phosphokinase (CK) and its isoenzymes and amylase.

c) Renal function: Blood urea nitrogen (BUN) and creatinine.

4. Hematology:

Blood samples are taken before and immediately after the surgery and every 4 hours during the preservation time for routine hematology study.

5. Coagulation factors:

Activated clotting time (ACT), fibrinogen, and prothrombin time.

6. Blood gas analysis:

Arterial and venous pH, pO_2, and pCO_2 measurements are performed before and immediately after the operation and every hour during the preservation period.

7. Urine output:

Recorded every hour.

8. Organ tissue wet/dry weight ratio:

Tissue samples are taken from the lungs every eight hours for wet/dry ratio determination. Tissue samples from all organs are taken at the end of preservation.

9. Pathology study:

Tissue samples are taken from the lungs every eight hours for EM study. Tissue samples are taken from other organs as needed during the preservation period and at the end of preservation.

BASIC INTERVENTIONS DURING THE PRESERVATION PERIOD

All interventions are directed at maintaining hemodynamic stability. Stable hemodynamics ensure that the organ block will survive for longer periods. The following parameters are important for maintaining a hemodynamically stable preparation.

1. Bath solution temperature:

The optimum temperature for this kind of preservation has not been extensively studied. We usually keep the bath temperature at approximately 32°C.

2. Respirator:

Any pressure- or volume-cycled respirator will work for the preparation. For dogs of 15 to 20 kg body weight, the following set-up has been used:
Tidal volume: 500-700 ml
Respirator rate: 10-20 rpm
PEEP: 4-8 cmH$_2$O
Gas mixture: 50% O_2 + 3% CO_2 + 47% N_2

3. Blood pressures:

Arterial systolic pressure: We have found that aortic systolic pressure in the range of 75-100 mmHg can maintain good organ function and will not cause excessive bleeding. Arterial pressure can be easily adjusted by transfusions of blood or plasma.

Arterial pulse pressure: Although it is not a simple matter to adjust pulse pressure, a pulse pressure of 40 to 50 mmHg usually indicates good organ function and adequate circulation.

Heart rate: The intrinsic heart rate in this preservation is usually in the range of 60-80 beats per minute. We do not pace the heart. Slower rates may occur at very low temperatures. A fast rate, combined with unstable hemodynamics, usually indicates some pathological condition. Immediate intervention and correction of the problem is required.

Central venous pressure: CVP should be the same as that found in the intact animal or slightly higher due to the disappearance of negative thoracic pressure. Unusually high CVP indicates either a kinked vena cava, decreased heart function, or both.

4. Arterial blood gas:

pH: When organs are functioning well, this value is maintained automatically. However, metabolic or respiratory acidosis may occur if arterial pressure is too low or if the respiratory setting is wrong.

$paCO_2$: When 3% CO_2 is used in the respirator, this value should be normal during preservation. Any change of gas mixture or respiratory setting can affect the value.

paO_2: If lung function is good, even room air can give a satisfactory paO_2. When 50% oxygen is used, paO_2 should be in the range of 250-280 mmHg. Lower paO_2 usually results from collapse of lung tissue, which occurs more easily due to the loss of negative pressure. It may be necessary to provide a "sigh," to increase inspiratory volume, or to use higher PEEP to correct lung collapse and prevent atelectasis.

5. Hematocrit:

Because the temperature used in our study is lower than normal body temperature, a lower hematocrit may be beneficial. We usually keep the hematocrit around 25%-40%. If the hematocrit is higher than 45%, plasma is given.

6. Blood chemistry:

It is necessary to administer potassium, calcium, and glucose by intravenous drip to maintain normal serum levels. If high urine output occurs, hypokalemia may result, and additional potassium supplementation may become necessary. Other electrolytes, such as sodium and chloride, are usually stable, and no special attention is needed. Due to the small blood volume, rapid infusion of any electrolyte can cause fluctuations in serum concentration and may result in organ damage. This is especially true for potassium.

7. Urine output:

In our studies, urine output is usually high at the beginning of preservation due to fluid infusions during harvesting. During the preservation period, urine output usually ranges from 5 to 50 ml per hour and can be adjusted by fluid infusion.

8. Intravenous administration:

This is another area where more research is needed. We use, in our experiments, only a basic formula to supplement very necessary elements. Drugs can be added for additional effects. In our experiments, four infusion groups are given:

a) Electrolytes: potassium (0.5 g/L) and calcium (1 g/L)

b) Nutrient: glucose (5%)

c) Antibiotics: ampicillin (1 g/L) and Flagyl (500 mg/L)

d) Diuretics: mannitol (12.5 g/L)

9. Intravenous injection:

The following injections are administrated every 2 hours:

a) Methylprednisolone (30 mg)

b) A fat emulsion, Soyacal (2 ml)

TECHNICAL PROBLEMS DURING HARVESTING AND PRESERVATION

1. Selection of experimental animals.

We have tried several animal species for our studies. Dogs were used first. Overall the results were good, with one exception: the dog liver is very sensitive to any form of stimulation. Liver congestion begins early and persists during the preservation period. This phenomenon is believed to be related to spasm of the hepatic vein sphincters.[1-3] Venous spasm is not as severe in pigs or humans. In our experience, liver congestion is not a major problem in Yorkshire pigs. However, pig lungs seem to be very fragile. A short period of high pressure on the respirator, such as when trying to expand a collapsed lobe after surgery, may damage the lungs and even burst an already expanded lung. Such damage can result in continuous air leaking and bleeding.

Small animals such as guinea pigs have also been tried. The operating time is short (less than half an hour), and fewer clamps are needed to remove the whole organ system.

Rabbits have been used by others in similar studies.[4-6] However, small animals do not provide enough blood for use in our detailed laboratory tests (20-30 ml of blood at each sampling period is needed for complete blood chemistry and hematology studies). Presently, we are using dogs for our studies, with the application of some drugs to alleviate liver congestion. The overall results are good. Dogs are large enough to provide sufficient blood samples for laboratory tests, an exercise which is essential for monitoring such a complicated preparation. Surgical time tends to be longer for a fat dog because much time is spent dissecting the fat tissue. We prefer a dog of moderate size (15-20 kg) with a relatively lean body. Some species, such as Newfoundland dogs, have large amount of body fat, and their lungs are more fragile. Avoidance of this type of animal appears prudent.

2. Correct alignment of the organs.

The abdominal organs, especially the liver and kidneys, are subject to torsion, and vascular occlusion can occur when the organs are removed because they are attached to the circulation only by the descending aorta and the inferior vena cava. When the organ block is placed in the bath chamber, the lungs float while the liver sinks. This causes torsion of the vena cava with resultant venous congestion, manifested by a drop in arterial blood pressure, swelling of the liver and decrease in urine output. Inotropic drugs usually do not help in this situation. Using some type of stand for the liver and kidneys while the organ block is in the water bath and adjusting the water level so that the organs are aligned in the same plane will reduce or eliminate the problem.

3. Special problems with the liver.

Because of its bulky size and rapid metabolism, the liver is quite vulnerable to mechanical or ischemic damage. Early studies have indicated that the liver is second only to the brain in vulnerability to ischemic damage.[7,8] Our experience has been that when dogs are used, if no special treatment is applied, liver damage could occur during the preservation period. The liver becomes visibly congested, the color darkens, and lymph exudes. Laboratory tests indicate liver injury as evidenced by an increase in liver-related enzymes such as AST, ALT, LDH, etc. Liver congestion can begin as early as the beginning of abdominal surgery.[9] The problem is probably related to the special anatomical structure of the hepatic veins, which differs from that of most other veins. Hepatic vein muscle is relatively well developed and lies chiefly in adventitia. This arrangement of the muscle permits the veins to play a role in controlling the hepatic circulation.[1] In an intact animal, hepatic congestion can be induced by a number of substances, such as extracts of Ascaris suum and hydatid cyst fluid, and is accompanied by severe shock, as evidenced by an extreme decrease in arterial blood pressure and even death of the animal if the dose of the substance is sufficiently large. That the cause of death was liver related was shown by the fact that hepatectomized dogs were little affected by doses that proved lethal for dogs with an intact liver.[10,11] One study has shown that the mechanism of liver congestion is a diffuse spasm of the entire hepatic venous side of the vasculature of the liver. This mechanism appears to be very important in dogs. However, it has also been shown to be present, although to a much lesser degree, in cats, rats, and even humans.[11] Because of this mechanism, the portal circulation is extremely susceptible to infection and ischemia, which can result in contraction of the hepatic vein and subsequent obstruction of venous outflow.[12,13] Certain drugs, such as epinephrine, may prevent the spasm, but, if the constriction is severe, it is difficult to eliminate.[14-16] However, several chemicals used in our laboratory have been shown to eliminate the constriction satisfactorily. This issue will be discussed later.

4. Nutritional supplies during the preservation period.

Longevity in the autoperfusion preparation is not limited only by the availability of oxygen. Metabolic factors are important. As much as 5% of myocardial adenosine 5'-triphosphate and phosphocreatine is consumed per cardiac cycle, and stored glycogen and triglycerides are able to maintain function for no longer than 6-12 minutes.[17] In isolated organs, bicarbonate content can fall rapidly as a result of lactic acid production by blood or by the liver. A liver, rich in glycogen, can produce much lactate when exposed to stress. Lactic acid accumulation then produces severe acidosis.[18] Normally, the main substrate for respiration in heart, liver and kidney is fat in the form of free fatty acids.[17,19] With the onset of ischemia, glycolysis is known to provide the majority of energy, while the use of free fatty acids is suppressed.[20] The lung uses free fatty acids for oxidation and synthetic reactions leading to the synthesis of phospholipids.[21] Glucose is also used in lung metabolism.[21] The store of free fatty acids in the organs is very low, and the amounts present in blood plasma are also very low.[18] While the organs are isolated, the main sources of supply (the gut and adipose tissue) are removed. Additional nutrients must be given. The need for substrate enhancement in a working heart-lung model was recognized early. In nonfed autoperfused heart-lung preparations, free fatty acids were depleted first, followed by glucose depletion.[22] Infusion of a balanced substrate and electrolyte solution provides adequate short-term metabolic support without light microscope or transmission electron microscope evidence of structural damage after a mean perfusion time of 7.9 hours.[23,24] All these studies on substrate enhancement used a simpler model in which only the heart and lungs were included.[17,22-24] Uniform results have not been obtained, and almost all the substrate provision for the autoperfusion systems is empirically based. Theoretically, the inclusion of the liver, pancreas and kidneys in the multiorgan block preparation should make substrate supply simpler. The liver has the ability to control and build up a normal external environment when perfused with a semisynthetic medium. The liver sheds amino acids, lactate and pyruvate until concentrations in the perfusion medium approximate those of normal blood plasma.[18,25]

In our experiments, we use a relatively simple nutrient combination. Only dextran and fat emulsion are given. The fat emulsion (Soyacal) is supplemented every two hours for nutrient supply. However, when Soyacal is infused into the inferior vena cava, an amount of 2 ml every two hours appears to be excessive because the emulsion can still be seen in the plasma after two hours. We now routinely infuse the emulsion through the portal vein, which increases absorption. However, the whole area of optimum nutritional requirement and what kinds of substances should be given needs much further research.

5. Reduction of leukocytes during the preservation period.

In all our experiments, one finding has been constant: despite a stable RBC count, there is always a large reduction in leukocyte concentration. This could be related to several factors: 1) there is no bone marrow in the system to provide new leukocytes; 2) bacterial infection, if it occurs, can reduce the number of leukocytes; 3) sequestration of WBC in the lungs could reduce the concentration of leukocytes in the circulation. Sequestration of leukocytes in the lungs has been confirmed in pathological studies showing a large number of leukocytes trapped in the lungs after preservation. Other studies have shown that depletion of leukocytes in the circulation could improve lung tissue survival time during preservation.[26,27] Activation of the complement system plus neutrophils and free oxygen radicals could be a major source of injury to the lungs and other organs. This may lead to final organ deterioration.[28,29] Studies related to this issue have not been performed and further experiments are needed.

6. Tissue damage during organ harvesting.

We have found that the length of the operation is related to the overall survival of the organs. If the operation is performed quickly and carefully, the organs usually survive longer and maintain good physiologic function. If the operation is done slowly, however, hypotension may result before the organ block is removed from the body, with resultant signs of deterioration in the lungs and liver. The lungs are most vulnerable because they dry out from exposure to the air. Surface damage thus created appears to accelerate throughout the preservation period. Long harvesting times will also result in excessive bleeding and/or fluid exudation, which will reduce circulating volume, causing further tissue damage. The most critical portion of the operation is dissecting the descending aorta. To detach the intercostal arteries, the heart and left lung must be pushed to the right, a maneuver that can collapse the lungs and distort blood vessels, resulting in hypotension. We suggest the prodigious use of surgical staplers, which can speed up dissection and reduce hemodynamic disturbance. The use of two surgical teams, one to carry out the abdominal dissection and another to dissect the chest, will greatly accelerate the harvesting time. The lungs should be covered with moistened towels during the chest operation.

7. Blood volume and hematocrit adjustments.

Adding the liver to the system appears to improve hemodynamic stability substantially. Even though the dissection is extensive during harvesting, very rarely does excessive bleeding persist during preservation. On the other hand, large doses of heparin have been administered to prevent clotting in some experiments.[30] An effective clotting mechanism is probably related to the normal production of clotting factors by a functioning liver. Any blood and plasma lost during the preservation period must be replaced to maintain physiologic perfusion of the organs. Because the lymph drainage of the abdominal organs is disrupted, lymph loss becomes a major component of volume depletion. Lymph flow from the abdominal lymphatic vessels may reach over 100 ml per hour at the beginning but will gradually decrease. The loss of lymph can result in high hematocrit levels, which are unfavorable in mild hypothermia. We usually infuse plasma when the hematocrit becomes elevated.

8. Preservable organs.

The basic organs in this multiorgan preparation include the heart, lungs, liver and kidneys. These organs are vital to the stability of the system because each has a unique function essential to maintaining the physiologic stability of the system. Other tissues or or-

gans can be added or removed without a major effect on survival. For example, the brain can be added to the system for preservation if necessary. The unique ability of the system to maintain continuous circulation during harvesting provides the only possibility for brain preservation. In this preservation procedure, the pancreas and duodenum are extirpated together with the other organs. This facilitates the collection of both bile and pancreatic secretions. The intestine itself probably does not contribute to the overall survival of the preparation and could possibly increase the risk of contamination. Whether it is necessary to include the intestine and the pancreas in studies of this nature is presently unclear.

RESULTS OF PRELIMINARY DOG STUDIES

In preliminary preservation experiments, using five adult mongrel dogs ranging in weight from 19-26 kg, the organ block survived from 9-25 hours, with an average survival time of 12.5 hours.

Cardiac function was well maintained. Aortic systolic pressure (AOSP) ranged from 75-125 mmHg, central venous pressure (CVP) from 0-5 mmHg, and portal venous pressure from 0-3 mmHg.

Alveolar ventilation and diffusion capacities were well maintained during the preservation period, as shown by arterial oxygen tension (paO_2), carbon dioxide tension ($paCO_2$) and A-a O_2 difference. A tidal volume of 500-700 mmHg with 4-8 cm H_2O PEEP maintained blood gases at normal levels and pH in the normal range. When 50% O_2 and 3% CO_2 were used, paO_2 was maintained at approximately 300 mmHg and $paCO_2$ at approximately 35 mmHg.

Bile output ranged from 5-20 ml/hour. The liver was the only organ that showed evidence of deterioration. Liver edema started to occur at the beginning of abdominal dissection. Diffuse darkening of tissue and severe sweating of the liver could be seen during dissection. Laboratory tests for liver function showed evidence of liver damage, including increased AST, ALT, CK, LDH, uric acid, etc.

The pancreas and duodenum showed normal color and size in most of the dogs. When the liver was congested, these organs also showed some congestion, but it was less severe than that of the liver. Secretions from these organs were constant even when bile output was decreased. Blood amylase levels increased immediately after the operation and then decreased to almost normal at 12 hours postoperatively. This indicated that damage was probably the result of surgical trauma and not of the preservation procedure.

Urine output ranged from 10-70 ml per hour with an average for each animal of 20.65 ml/hour; this output was much higher than that expected for a normal animal of this weight. The kidneys showed normal size and color during preservation. In the longest surviving system, the kidney showed some swelling after 16 hours, and urine output decreased. In one system in which the inferior vena cava was kinked, the kidneys showed a dark color with subsequent hematuria. In most experiments, urinalysis indicated normal kidney function and urine composition. A typical urinalysis result is shown in Table 1. Blood creatinine levels were significantly lower following removal of the organs from the body ($p < 0.01$).

RBC concentrations were maintained in the normal range throughout the study and were easily adjusted by blood or plasma transfusion when necessary. However, WBC counts showed a continuous and significant decrease during the preservation period ($p < 0.005$). Blood platelet levels also showed some decrease during the preservation period.

Potassium infusions were given to maintain normal serum potassium levels. Sodium levels were slightly higher than normal but still within normal limits. Calcium, glucose, and osmolarity were maintained within normal limits in most of the experiments.

Fibrinogen levels and prothrombin times were normal during the preservation period. Activated clotting time (ACT) was measured in some experiments and was also within normal limits.

Microscopic studies suggested good tissue preservation. At 12 hours, lung sections showed normal structure and no evidence of

Table 1. A typical report of urinalysis

Color: Pale yellow

Specific gravity: 1.3

pH: 8

Protein: Trace

Glucose: 2+

Ketones: 0

Bilirubin: 0

Blood: 1+

RBC: 5-10/HPF

WBC: 1-3/HPF

Epith cells: 0-3/HPF

Casts: 0/LPF

Potassium: 11 /L

Protein 20 mg/dl

Calcium: 4.2 meq/L

Osmolality: 378 mOsm/kg

edema. Mononuclear macrophages, some with cytoplasmic pigment, appeared focally clustered around terminal bronchioles. Myocardium of the left ventricle showed focal edema. The liver showed some focal congestion of sinusoids around the central vein accompanied by microdroplet fatty change in centrizonal hepatocytes.

In summary, the use of this autoperfusion multiorgan block preparation as a new method for preserving major organs is a fruitful area for research. The simplicity of the preoperative preparation and the possibility that physiologic functions can be monitored in the preservation process provide a unique opportunity for study. The natural circulation and physiologic environment allow for the possibility of long-term multiorgan preservation. The liver congestion seen in the dog studies may not be as severe in other animals or in humans. Methods for preventing or alleviating congestion during the preservation period so that longer preservation times are possible will be discussed in the next two chapters.

APPENDIX

System Malfunctions and Possible Causes During Preservation

The organ block contains six major organs of the body. If one organ is damaged, the other organs will be affected due to the interaction among the organs. If a key organ is malfunctioning, the whole system will be jeopardized. Because the organ block is much smaller than a whole body, less buffer is present in the system. A small mistake may not harm a whole body but may cause severe damage to the organ block. For example, a small air bubble flushed into an arterial line in the femoral artery will be flushed to the peripheral circulation of the leg, resulting in no destruction because of collateral circulation. However, a bubble injected into an arterial line placed in the descending aorta may destroy a kidney, because there is no other way for the bubble to escape from the system. If proper interventions are made, the system should be very stable and maintain normal function for a long period of time. However, when an emergency occurs, the organ block should be treated with life-threatening consideration. The following disturbances have been seen in our preliminary studies; possible causes of such disturbances and prevention measures are presented.

I. HYPOTENSION

During the preservation period, arterial systolic pressure should be approximately 100 mmHg, and no special drugs are needed to maintain the pressure if all the organs are functioning normally. If hypotension occurs, there must be some problem, and immediate attention is required to correct the abnormality.

A. Possible Causes
1. Bleeding in the system.
2. Blood transfusion is too slow to match volume loss.
3. Severe acidosis (respiratory or metabolic).
4. Severe liver congestion.
5. Hypoxia.
6. Hypocalcemia.
7. Hypokalemia or hyperkalemia.
8. Severe hypothermia (bath solution temperature too low).
9. Severe infection.
10. Deteriorated heart function.
11. Severe arrhythmia (usually results from hypokalemia, acidosis, hypoxia and deteriorated heart function).
12. Mechanical problems (clotted line, drifted zero, etc.).

B. Prevention
1. Maintaining careful hemostasis.
2. Giving generous blood transfusions to maintain circulatory volume.
3. Preventing and correcting acidosis.
4. Avoiding and correcting hypoxia.
5. Maintaining blood electrolytes at normal levels.
6. Using aseptic technique and antibiotics.
7. Maintaining stable temperature.

II. ACID-BASE DISTURBANCE

During normal preservation, there is very little chance of developing acidosis or alkalosis. According to our experience, early acid-base disturbance is of respiratory origin resulting from an incorrect setting of the respirator. An incorrect gas mixture or hyper- or hypo-ventilation can shift the acid-base balance. Because the lungs are outside the chest cage, the physiologic negative pressure does not exist, which makes it easier for the lungs to be over- or underinflated. Inspection of the lungs can reveal the cause of the problem. In the later stages of the experiments, acid-base disturbance is usually metabolic, resulting from loss or deterioration in organ function.

A. Possible causes of acidosis
1. Hypoventilation.
2. Atelectasis.
3. Low oxygen concentration in the gas mixture.
4. High carbon dioxide concentration.
5. Excessive dead space.
6. Deteriorating heart function.
7. Deteriorating lung function.

B. Management
1. Checking gas mixture to make sure that there is enough gas and that the gas mixture is correct.

2. Checking the respirator to make sure the dead space is correct and all the connections are intact. Placing the organ block in a bath tank tends to increase the length of respirator tubing, and connections become vulnerable to becoming loose and disconnected. Readjusting the respirator may be necessary to suit the organ block. Tidal volume is determined by the body weight of the donor animal rather than by the weight of the organ block.
3. Checking the lungs to see if lobes are collapsed. Reexpanding the lungs will eliminate any atelectasis.
4. Checking to see if the organs are correctly aligned. In particular, the inferior vena cava between the liver and the heart should not be stretched or kinked. The kidneys must not become twisted in the bath solution.
5. Giving an appropriate dose of sodium bicarbonate if metabolic acidosis is present.

III. PREMATURE RENAL FAILURE

A. POSSIBLE CAUSES

1. Obstruction of renal artery or vein.
   a) Inferior vena cava obstruction caused by improper alignment.
   b) Severe liver congestion.
   c) Clot or air emboli in the renal artery.
   d) Clot formation in the renal vein or inferior vena cava.
   e) Rotation of the kidney in the water bath.
2. Severe acidosis.
3. Severe hemolysis.
4. Long-time ischemia caused by hypotension during harvesting or preservation.
5. Drug-induced damage to the kidneys.
6. Severe infection.
7. Increased renal vascular resistance during preservation.

B. PREVENTION

1. Avoiding any clots or air in the arterial line.
2. Aligning the organs properly so that the inferior vena cava is not kinked.
3. Keeping the kidneys in the correct posi-

tion in the water bath. Kinks or stretches to the renal artery or vein must be avoided.
4. Keeping arterial pressure normal.
5. Using appropriate doses of drugs.
6. Performing the operation under sterile conditions.
7. Preventing acidosis.
8. Using appropriate blood type to reduce hemolysis.
9. Using antibiotics.
10. Administering fluids to maintain urine flow.

IV. PULMONARY EDEMA

A. POSSIBLE CAUSES

1. Lung ischemia from long-time hypotension.
2. Mechanical injury induced during the operation.
3. Insufficient lung expansion.
4. Allergic reaction (blood, drugs, etc.).
5. Bacterial contamination during the operation or preservation period.
6. Fluid retention caused by renal failure.
7. Water and sodium over-transfusion.
8. Severely diluted blood.
9. Low plasma protein.
10. Air or clot emboli induced from venous lines.
11. Loss of heart function.

B. PREVENTION

1. Maintaining normal systemic pressure.
2. Keeping the lungs properly inflated during preservation.
3. Avoiding mechanical injury during operation.
4. Maintaining careful hemostasis to reduce blood transfusion.
5. Performing all procedures under sterile conditions.
6. Protecting the kidney.
7. Limiting sodium transfusion during preservation.
8. Avoiding over-transfusion of fluids.
9. Avoiding the use of severely diluted blood.
10. Moistening lung surfaces to avoid drying out.
11. Using antibiotics.
12. Avoiding air or clots in the venous line.

REFERENCES

1. Gibson JB: The hepatic veins in man and their sphincter mechanisms. J Anat Lond 1959; 93:369-379.

2. Walker WF, MacDonald JS, Pickard C: Hepatic vein sphincter mechanism in the dog. Br J Surg 1960; 48:218-220.

3. Moreno AH, Rousselot LM, Burchell AR, Bono RF, Burke JH: Studies on the outflow tracts of the liver: II. On the outflow tracts of the canine liver with particular reference to its regulation by the hepatic vein sphincter mechanisms. Ann Surg 1962; 155:427-433.

4. Segel LD, Ensunsa JL, Boyle WA 3rd: Prolonged support of working rabbit hearts using fluosol-43 or erythrocyte media. Am J Physiol 1987; 252:H349-H359.

5. Muskett A, Burton NA, Grossman M, Gay WA Jr: The rabbit autoperfusion heart-lung preparation. J Surg Res 1988; 44:104-108.

6. Muskett AD, Burton NA, Gay WA Jr, Miller M, Rabkin MS: Preservation in the rabbit autoperfusion heart-lung preparation: a potential role for indomethacin. Surg Forum 1986; 37:252-254.

7. Harris KA, Wallace AC, Wall WJ: Tolerance of the liver to ischemia in the pig. J Surg Res 1982; 33:524-530.

8. Lambotte L: Liver preservation. In: Toledo-Pereyra LH, ed. Basic Concepts of Organ Procurement, Perfusion, and Preservation. New York: Academic Press, 1982:225-257.

9. Chien S, Todd EP, Diana JN, O'Connor WN: A simple technique for multiorgan preservation. J Thorac Cardiovasc Surg 1988; 95: 55-61.

10. Grana A, Mann FC, Essex HE: Influence of the liver on the shock produced by extracts of certain parasites. Am J Physiol 1947; 148:243-252.

11. Thomas WD, Essex HE: Observations on the hepatic venous circulation with special reference to the sphincteric mechanism. Am J Physiol 1949; 158:303-310.

12. Calne RY: Preservation of the liver. In: Calne RY, ed. Liver Transplantation. New York: Grune & Stratton, 1983:17-23.

13. Ritchie HD, Hardcastle JD: Liver. In: Ritchie HD, Hardcastle JD, eds. Isolated Organ Perfusion. London: University Park Press, 1973:71-134.

14. Deysach LJ: The nature and location of the "sphincter mechanism" in the liver as determined by drug actions and vascular injections. Am J Physiol 1941; 132:713-724.

15. Andrews WHH, Hecker R, Maegraith BG, Ritchie HD: The action of adrenaline, L-noradrenaline, acetylcholine and other substances on the blood vessels of the perfused canine liver. J Physiol (London) 1955; 128:413-434.

16. Andrews WHH, Hecker R, Maegraith BG: The actyion of adrenaline, noradrenaline, acetylcholine and histamine on the perfused liver of the monkey, cat and rabbit. J Physiol (London) 1956; 132:509-521.

17. Riveron FA, Ross JH, Schwartz KA, et al: Energy expenditure of autoperfusion heart-lung preparation. Circulation 1988; 78 (Suppl. III):103-109.

18. Krebs HA: Metabolic requirements of isolated organs. Transplant Proc 1974; 6:237-239.

19. Vik-Mo H, Mjos OD: Influence of free fatty acids on myocardial oxygen consumption and ischemic injury. Am J Cardiol 1981; 48:361-365.

20. Hudon MPJ, Jamieson WRE, Qayumi AK, Dougan H, Sartori C, Lyster DM: Assessment of myocardial metabolic state after hypothermic heart preservation for transplantation utilizing radioiodinated free fatty acid imaging. J Heart Lung Transplant 1991; 10:704-709.

21. Felts JM: Biochemistry of the lung. Health Phys 1964; 10:973-979.

22. Robicsek F, Masters TN, Duncan GD, Denyer MH, Rise HE, Etchison M: An autoperfused heart-lung-preparation: metabolism and function. Heart Transplant 1985; 4:334-338.

23. Stewart RW, Morimoto T, Golding LR, Harasaki H, Olsen E, Nose Y: Canine heart-lung autoperfusion. Trans Am Soc Artif Int Organs 1985; 31:206-210.

24. Kontos GJ, Borkon AM, Baumgartner WA et al: Improved myocardial and pulmonary preservation by metabolic substrate enhancement in the autoperfused working heart-lung preparation. J Heart Transplant 1988; 7:140-144.

25. Guyton AG: Physiology of the human body. 5th ed. Philadelphia: W. B. Saunders Co., 1979.397-424.

26. Hall TS, Breda MA, Baumgartner WA, et al: The role of leukocyte depletion in reducing injury to the lung after hypothermic ischemia. Curr Surg 1987; 44:137-139.

27. Naka Y, Hirose H, Matsuda H, et al: Prevention of pulmonary edema in autoperfusing heart-lung preparation by FUT-175 and leukocyte depletion. Transplant Proc 1989; 21:1353-1356.

28. Clark IA: Tissue damage caused by free oxygen radicals. Pathology 1986; 18:181-186.

29. Ward PA, Till GO, Kunkel R, Beauchamp C: Evidence for role of hydroxyl radical in complement and neutrophil-dependent tissue injury. J Clin Invest 1983; 72:789-801.

30. Chien S, Diana JN, Oeltgen PR, Todd EP, O'Connor WN: Eighteen to 37 hours' preservation of major organs using a new autoperfusion multiorgan preparation. Ann Thorac Surg 1989; 47:860-867.

CHAPTER 4

EXTENDING ORGAN SURVIVAL TIME USING HIBERNATION INDUCTION TRIGGER

In this chapter, we report the preliminary results of our experiments with using plasma from deeply hibernating woodchucks (*Marmota monax*), which contains hibernation induction trigger (HIT), in the multiorgan block preparation.

MATERIAL AND METHODS

SAMPLE PROCUREMENT

Plasma assayed for HIT activity was obtained from woodchucks weighing 3-5 kg. The animals were maintained at $4°$-$6°C$ during the winter months in a hibernaculum. Blood was drawn aseptically by intraventricular puncture while each animal was in deep hibernation, as evidenced by a core temperature of approximately $5°C$ and a heart rate ranging from 1-2 beats per minute. Normally, it required 1-2 hours for full arousal to occur after blood collection. During this time core temperature slowly rose to $37°C$ and heart rate to its normal homeothermic baseline level. The whole blood was placed in heparinized tubes and centrifuged to obtain plasma, which was then frozen at $-70°C$ for later use.

ANIMALS STUDIED

Twenty adult mongrel dogs weighing 17-30 kg each were used in this study. The study group (Group 1) consisted of 12 dogs that received HIT-containing plasma before and after the operation. The control group (Group 2) consisted of 8 dogs that received the same amount of saline but no HIT. To obtain normal organ wet/dry weight ratios, tissue samples from the heart, lungs, liver, pancreas, duodenum and kidney were taken from fifteen normal dogs and used for comparison.

Group 1 animals were further divided into two subgroups. For group 1A (6 dogs), the organ block was preserved as long as the organs were functioning. For Group 1B (6 dogs), the left lungs were transplanted after more than 24 hours of preservation.

All animals received humane care in compliance with the "Principles of Laboratory Animal Care" formulated by the National Society for Medical Research and the "Guide for the Care and Use of Laboratory Animals" published by the National Institutes of Health (NIH Publication No. 85-23, revised 1985).

PRETREATMENT

All dogs were given neomycin (2 gm orally once a day) for three days before surgery to sterilize their digestive systems. The dogs were fasted for five hours prior to surgery. They were then anesthetized, and 10 ml of plasma containing HIT from deeply hibernating woodchucks was injected intravenously into each dog in the study group two hours prior to the operation. Normal saline (10 ml) was given to dogs in the control group.

SURGICAL TECHNIQUE

The technique used in this study was the same as that described in Chapter 3.

INTERVENTIONS

The temperature of the preserved organ block was maintained at 32°C by heating the water bath with a constant temperature circulator. Artificial respiration was maintained with a Harvard volume-cycled respirator at a tidal volume of 500-700 ml, a rate of 10-20 rpm, and PEEP of 2-6 cm H_2O. A gas mixture of 50% O_2 + 3% CO_2 + 47% N_2 was utilized. A 5% dextrose solution containing the following drugs was infused through the portal vein at 10-20 ml/hour: dextrose (5%), calcium chloride (1 g/L), insulin (50 units/L), mannitol (12.5 g/L), methylprednisolone (500 mg/L), penicillin (1,000,000 units/L) and Flagyl (500 mg/L). A separate 5% dextrose solution containing potassium chloride (0.5 g/L) was infused slowly through the portal vein to maintain serum potassium at a normal level.

A fat emulsion (Soyacal, 2 ml) and methylprednisolone (30 mg) were injected through the portal vein every two hours. Blood transfusions were given to maintain aortic systolic pressure at 75-100 mmHg and central venous pressure (CVP) at 0-10 mmHg. Plasma was given instead of whole blood if the hematocrit was higher than 45%.

INFUSION OF WOODCHUCK PLASMA DURING PRESERVATION

In the study group, 4 ml of plasma containing HIT was infused through the portal vein every four hours during the preservation period. In the control group, 4 ml of normal saline was infused at the same intervals during the preservation period.

MONITORING

Aortic pressure, left ventricular pressure and dp/dt, central venous pressure, portal venous pressure, and heart rate were monitored and recorded on a Gould multichannel recorder (Gould, Inc., Centerville, OH) throughout the preservation period. Aortic flow was measured with a Transonic dual-channel flowmeter (Transonic Systems, Inc., Ithaca, NY). Temperature, urine output, bile production, and duodenal and pancreatic secretions were collected and recorded every hour. Visible changes, including color, size, and bleeding for each organ, respiratory pressure, tidal volume, and PEEP for the lungs, were recorded every hour. Arterial blood gas and hematocrit measurements were taken before the operation and every hour during the preservation period using an IL Blood Gas-Electrolyte Analyzer (Instrumentation Laboratory, Lexington, MA). Venous blood samples were taken before the operation and every four hours during the preservation period. These were used for hematological and blood chemistry measurements, which included lactic acid tests and heart, liver, pancreas and kidney function tests. In Group 1A, tissue samples were taken from the lungs every eight hours for lung tissue wet/dry weight ratios and electron microscope studies. At the termination of the study, specimens were taken from each organ for wet/dry weight ratios and pathologic examinations.

DETERMINATION OF TISSUE WET/DRY WEIGHT RATIO

Tissue samples used for wet/dry weight ratio measurements were blotted to remove

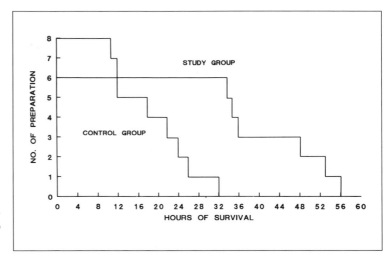

Fig. 1. Comparison of survival times between Group 1A and the control group.

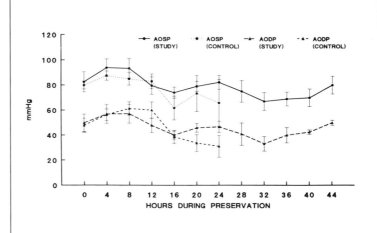

Fig. 2. Changes in aortic systolic pressures (AOSP) and aortic diastolic pressures (AODP) in the two groups during the preservation period. (Values are mean ± SEM.)

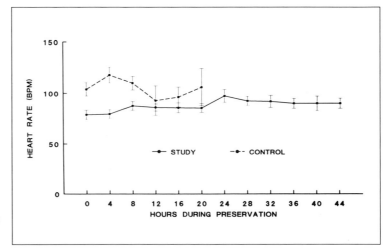

Fig. 3. Heart rate changes during preservation.

excess fluid, and wet weight was measured. The dry weight was determined after the samples had been in an oven at 85°C for 72 hours.

STATISTICAL ANALYSIS

All laboratory test results obtained before the operation (blood gases, hematocrit, blood chemistries, hematology, lactic acid and enzymes for heart, liver, pancreas and kidney functions) were used as normal controls. These controls were compared to the results obtained during the preservation period. Heart function and urine output were measured immediately after harvesting and during the preservation period, and these results were compared. Tissue wet/dry weight ratios for all organs were compared with those obtained from normal dogs.

For comparisons within a group, ANOVA and Student-Newman-Keuls tests were used to compare the data obtained every four hours during the preservation period with those obtained preoperatively. If a comparison was needed between the study group and the control group at a certain point, ANOVA and unpaired Student *t*-tests were used. All data are expressed as mean ± standard error of the mean, with statistical significance assigned at p<0.05.

ORGAN FUNCTION DURING THE PRESERVATION PERIOD

The mean survival time of the organs in group 1A was 43.4 ± 4.1 hours and ranged from 33.5-56 hours. In the control group, the survival time ranged from 9-31 hours, with an average of 16.2 ± 2.6 hours. (p<0.001, Fig. 1) Blood or plasma transfusions were given during the preservation period. The amount of blood or plasma used ranged from 900-3200 ml, with an hourly blood or plasma transfusion rate of 33-100 ml.

CARDIAC FUNCTION

In the study group, aortic pressures and heart rate were stable during the preservation period. Aortic systolic pressure, which ranged from 67 ± 8 to 94 ± 7 mmHg, was easily adjusted by blood or plasma transfusions. No inotropic drug administrations were required. Aortic diastolic pressure ranged from 33 ± 6 to 57 ± 8 mmHg. Aortic pulse pressure ranged from 28 ± 6 to 37 ± 4 mmHg and did not fluctuate appreciably during the preservation period. (Immediately after the operation it was 33 ± 3 mmHg; at 44 hours it was 30 ± 7 mmHg. Fig. 2) The heart rate ranged from 80 ± 5 to 97 ± 6 beats per minute. The heart rate was related to the temperature of the bath solution. When the temperature was lower than 30°C, the heart rate decreased. (Fig. 3) Mean CVP was 2.9 ± 0.7 mmHg at the beginning of preservation and increased slightly to 8.8 ± 2.3 mmHg at 40 hours. (Fig. 4) Mean left ventricular maximum dp/dt was 1168 ± 88 mmHg/second at the beginning of preservation. It increased to 1618

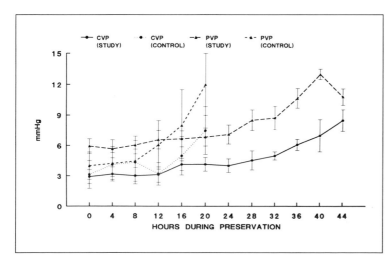

Fig. 4. (Left) Changes in central venous pressure (CVP) and portal venous pressure (PVP) in the two groups during preservation.

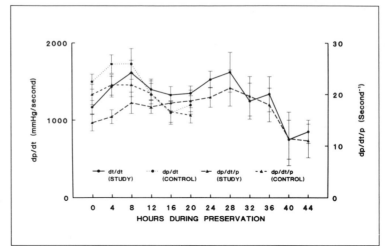

Fig. 5. Left ventricular dt/dt and dp/dt/p in the two groups during preservation.

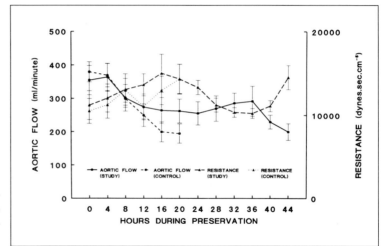

Fig. 6. Blood flow in the descending aorta and calculated systemic resistance during preservation.

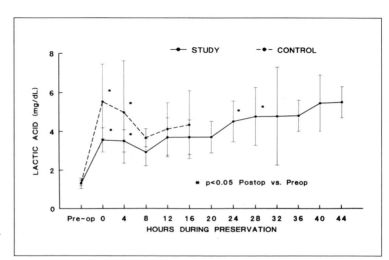

Fig. 7. Serum lactic acid levels during preservation.

± 162 mmHg/second after 8 hours and remained stable until 32-36 hours, then decreased gradually to 1340 ± 228 mmHg/second after 36 hours and to 850 ± 150 mmHg/second at 44 hours. Mean left ventricular dp/dt/p was 14.5 ± 1.6 (second^{-1}) at the beginning of preservation. It increased to 18.4 ± 2.1 (second^{-1}) at 8 hours, then remained at or above this level for up to 36 hours. It decreased slightly to 11.1 ± 3.3 (second^{-1}) at 44 hours. (Fig. 5) Blood flow in the descending aorta ranged from 256 ± 37 ml/min to 365 ± 41 ml/min and tended to decrease after 40 hours. Calculated systemic resistance ranged from 10232 ± 511 (dynes•sec•cm^{-5}) to 15039 ± 1967 (dynes.sec. cm^{-5}) and tended to increase after 40 hours of preservation. (Fig. 6) The average serum lactic acid level was 1.3 ± 0.3 mMol/L before surgery. It increased gradually during the preservation period and averaged 5.5 ± 01.5 mMol/L at 40 hours. (Fig. 7) Both total creatine phosphokinase (CK) and CK-MB increased during the preservation period. (Fig. 8) Heart function deteriorated 1-4 hours before overall system failure occurred.

In the organ blocks treated with HIT-containing plasma, the heart was very sensitive to hyperkalemia. In the study group, all deaths occurring before 48 hours were caused by hyperkalemia, which resulted from potassium over-transfusion. Sudden cardiac arrest occurred in three experiments when blood potassium levels increased above 6 mMol/L, even though all organs appeared to be in good functional condition.

In the control group, heart function was also well maintained during the preservation period, although the survival time was much shorter than that of the study group.

Lung Function

Tidal volume was maintained from 500-700 ml for the dogs used in this study during the preservation period. The maximum respiratory pressure ranged from 8-22 mmHg. Lung function was well maintained within 36 hours. When a gas mixture of 50% O_2 + 3% CO_2 + 47% N_2 was used during the preservation period, arterial oxygen tension ranged from 201 ± 42 to 326 ± 14 mmHg and carbon dioxide tension ranged from 21 ± 2 to 33 ± 3 mmHg. Arterial pH values ranged from 7.33 ± 0.02 to 7.45 ± 0.03. These parameters did not change appreciably within 36 hours. After that time, paO_2 and pH started to decrease, but $paCO_2$ remained at the same levels. (Fig. 9) Calculated airway resistance ranged from 0.012 ± 0.003 to 0.019 ± 0.004 mmHg/ml. This value increased to 0.024 ± 0.003 at 40 hours. Pulmonary vascular resistance ranged from 1908 ± 256 to 2641 ± 538 dynes•sec•cm^{-5} during the preservation period. This value was higher after 40 hours than at the beginning. (Fig. 10) Lung color changes started earlier than functional

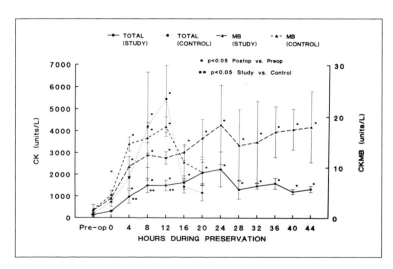

Fig. 8. (Right) Changes in serum creatine phosphokinase (CK) and CK-MB isoenzyme levels during preservation.

changes. The change of color was mainly related to exposure of the lungs' surfaces to air during harvesting. Lung tissue samples were studied by electron microscopy every four hours, and good tissue preservation was maintained for up to 32 hours (Fig. 11). Lung tissue wet/dry ratio was 5.45 ± 0.18 at the end of preservation, which was higher than that of normal dog lungs (4.91 ± 0.10, $p<0.025$).

In the control group, blood gases also remained normal for approximately 12 hours. Although paO_2 tended to be lower and $paCO_2$ tended to be higher than the values in the study group, the differences were not statistically significant. Lung color changes and lung deterioration occurred earlier in the control group than in the study group. Signs of deterioration included spot redness, patchy atelectasis and local edema.

The harvesting procedure can affect lung preservation time substantially. If the lung is damaged during harvesting, by extended exposure to air, for example, the damage will be carried on to the preservation time and the color change will not disappear. Instead, the damage will increase during preservation. Lung edema or even hemorrhage could occur at the damaged area. Any laceration of lung tissue will cause bleeding and air leaks. Protecting the lung tissue during the harvesting period is extremely important for a successful lung preservation.

LIVER FUNCTION

In the study group, bile output during the preservation period ranged from 1.4-5.9 ml per hour. The liver maintained good shape

Fig. 9. Changes in blood gas values during the preservation period. paO_2: Arterial oxygen tension. $paCO_2$: Arterial carbon dioxide tension.

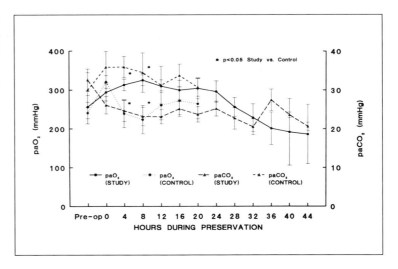

Fig. 10. Changes in maximum respiratory pressure and airway resistance during preservation.

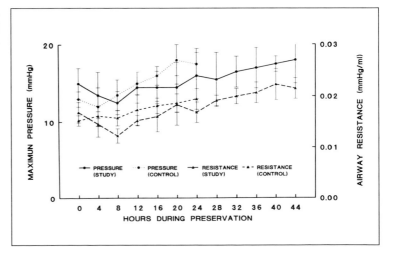

and function. Changes in liver-related enzyme levels reached a double peak during preservation. Both serum aspartate aminotransferase (AST) and alanine amino-transferase (ALT) increased immediately after harvesting, decreased during the preservation period, and tended to increase again after 36 hours. AST was 35 ± 4 units/L before surgery. It increased immediately to 249 ± 75 units/L after the surgery, decreased to 123 ± 15 at 12 hours, and then increased gradually after 20 hours. At 40 hours the AST level was 884 ± 520 units/L. ALT changes exhibited a similar pattern, but the late increase was not as severe as that of AST. (Fig. 12) The AST and ALT increases were not consistent. In some systems, the levels remained stable. However, in a few systems, the increase was severe. Mean serum lactic dehydrogenase (LDH) was 83 ± 24 U/L before the operation and increased to 242 ± 60 U/L at the beginning of the preservation period (p<0.05). It decreased to 121 ± 14 U/L at 8 hours and remained stable until 32 hours, then increased gradually to 416 ± 158 U/L at 40 hours. The level of LDH_5 isoenzyme, an indicator of hepatic congestion and liver injury, was 78 ± 34 U/L before the operation. It increased to 162 ± 49 U/L immediately after surgery and decreased to 38 ± 5 at 4 hours. It remained at this lower level during the preservation period, then increased to 132 ± 38 U/L at 40 hours. (Fig. 13) Serum alkaline phosphatase (ALP) level was 63 ± 9 U/L before the operation. It decreased to 31 ± 6 immediately after surgery and remained low during the preser-

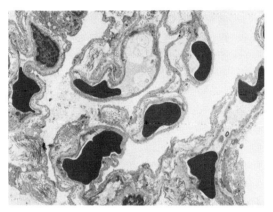 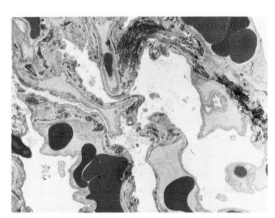

Fig. 11. Lung tissue electron microscope studies during preservation. The samples were taken every 4 hours. The samples shown here were taken at 16 and 32 hours during the preservation period.

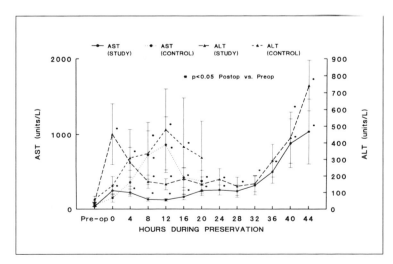

Fig. 12. Changes in serum aspartate amino-transferase (AST) and alanine amino-transferase (ALT) levels during the preservation period.

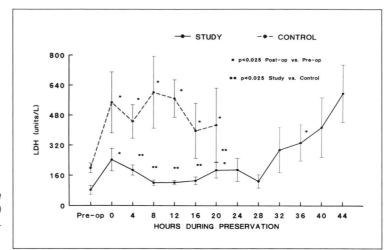

Fig. 13. Changes in serum lactic dehydrogenase (LDH) levels in the two groups during preservation.

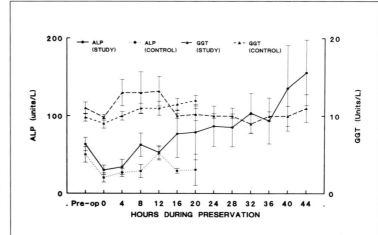

Fig. 14. Changes in serum alkaline phosphatase (ALP) and gamma glutamyl transpeptidase (GGT) levels during preservation.

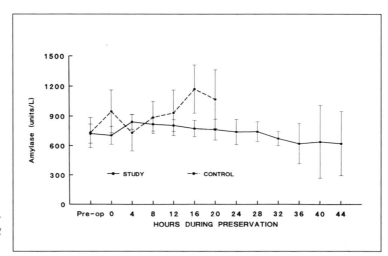

Fig. 15. Serum amylase levels in the two groups during preservation.

vation period. It increased slightly to 230 ± 92 U/L at 40 hours. The serum gamma glutamyl transpeptidase (GGT) level was very stable during the preservation period. It remained at the 10-12 U/L range throughout the preservation period (Fig. 14). Total bilirubin was 0.15 ± 0.02 mg/dL before the operation. It remained at 0.18 ± 0.04 to 0.39 ± 0.08 mg/dL during the preservation period. Bilirubin values were similar in the control group.

Distinct differences were found between the study group and the control group concerning liver preservation. In the study group, the liver usually retained its normal size, pink color and softness to the touch during the preservation period. In some experiments, the liver showed signs of congestion, including enlarged size, darkening surface and stiffness to the touch. However, these signs gradually disappeared and the liver returned to normal after HIT was infused. In the control group, the liver exhibited signs of congestion as soon as the abdominal operation began and deteriorated during preservation. The severity of liver congestion changed with time. Early signs included marked swelling, patchy darkening, stiffness to the touch, and continuous fluid exudation from the surface. The changes became worse as the preservation continued. After 12 hours, most of the livers were enlarged, pale, and stiff. Liver disturbance occurred in all experiments in the control group but at different severity levels. It occurred more severely or earlier in some experiments but less severely or later in others. Very severe liver congestion contributed to hypotension. Severe liver congestion caused early overall deterioration in four experiments. This change appeared to be caused by disturbance of liver circulation, because the liver might return to "normal" appearance after the circulation stopped. The increase of serum enzyme levels occurred earlier and was more severe in the control group. (Fig. 12)

Pancreatic and Duodenal Function

Changes in the pancreas and duodenum were mainly related to the patency of the portal vein rather than to the preservation itself. Since no anticoagulant was used, clot formation in the portal vein around the indwelling catheters could cause circulation disturbances in the pancreas and duodenum. In such cases, swelling and/or hemorrhage of the pancreas or duodenum might be seen. However, this happened only twice in the entire study group. In most experiments, the pancreas and duodenum exhibited minimal changes during the preservation period. Secretions from these organs ranged from 1.3-8.8 ml/hour (total 30-450 ml) and averaged 5.2 ml/hour. Average serum amylase level was 723 ± 92 units/L before the operation. It remained very stable, ranging from 620 ± 168 to 841 ± 71 units/L during the preservation period. (Fig. 15)

In the control group, serum amylase ranged from 731 ± 173 to 1170 ± 278 units/L during the preservation period. The pancreas and duodenum appeared congested when severe liver congestion occurred.

Renal Function

In the study group, total urine output ranged from 610-2400 ml during the preservation period and averaged 15-77 ml per hour, an elevated level for such a small tissue mass. (Fig. 16) Kidney function was well maintained during the preservation period. No excess water accumulated in the system. No premature renal failure occurred in the study group. Blood urea nitrogen (BUN) averaged 16.2 ± 1.5 mg/dL before surgery. It decreased to 5.8 ± 0.7 mg/dL at eight hours and remained at this low level throughout the preservation period ($p < 0.01$ at 32 hours). Serum creatinine averaged 0.9 ± 0.1 mg/dL before surgery. It decreased to 0.2 ± 0.03 mg/dL at 8 hours ($p < 0.001$) and remained at a relatively low level during preservation. ($p < 0.01$ at 32 hours, Fig. 17)

In the control group, total urine output ranged from 13-650 ml and from 0.6-54 ml per hour. Serum creatinine levels also decreased while the kidney was working. BUN decreased very little during preservation and was much higher than that of the study group ($p < 0.001$ at 16 hours). Premature renal failure occurred in two systems in the control group. Renal failure caused excess water retention, blood pH and electrolyte imbalances and eventual death.

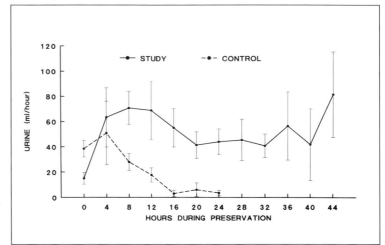

Fig. 16. Hourly urine output in two groups during preservation.

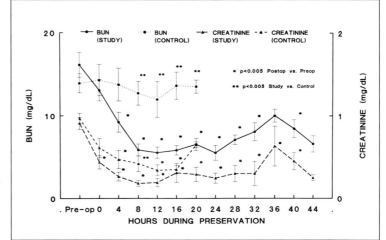

Fig. 17. Changes in blood urea nitrogen (BUN) and creatinine levels during the preservation period.

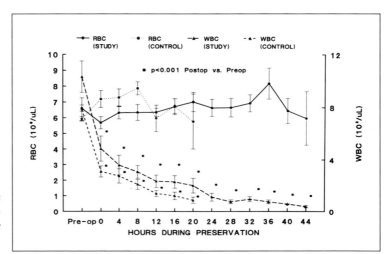

Fig. 18. Hematology studies during the preservation period. RBC: red blood cell; WBC: white blood cell.

HEMATOLOGY STUDY

In the study group, RBC concentrations were kept stable during the preservation period by blood or plasma transfusions. Heparin was not used, and bleeding was very minimal even though the dissection was extensive. The RBC count was 6.6 ± 0.2 (10^6/μL) before surgery. It ranged from 5.7 ± 0.4 to 8.2 ± 0.9 (10^6/μL) during the preservation period. Because of tissue cut, lymph exudation was prominent in the early preservation period. The RBC concentration tended to increase due to this lymph exudation. Plasma infusion was necessary in many experiments to prevent the development of a high hematocrit level. The WBC count was 11.34 ± 1.18 (10^3/μL) before surgery. It decreased to 3.05 ± 0.49 (10^3/μL) at 8 hours and continued to decrease to 0.57 ± 0.03 (10^3/μL) at 40 hours ($p < 0.001$, Fig. 18). Platelet levels decreased from 305 ± 32 (10^3/μL) before surgery to their lowest level of 122 ± 30 (10^3/μL) at 40 hours and were 127 ± 40 (10^3/μL) at 44 hours. (Fig. 19) Free plasma hemoglobin exhibited a two-fold increase at 24 hours in the study group.

In the control group, blood cell changes were similar to those in the study group. However, free plasma hemoglobin increased tenfold at eight hours, which was a more severe change than that found in the study group. (Fig. 20)

Blood cell levels usually decreased immediately after harvesting due to blood loss and to the fact that only crystalloid infusions were given during surgery. Blood or plasma transfusions were given after the organ block was placed in the bath solution, and this increased blood cell levels gradually.

BLOOD COAGULATION FACTORS

Serum fibrinogen ranged from 100-250 mg% and remained stable during the preservation period. Plasma prothrombin time ranged from 12-30 seconds. It increased slightly during the preservation time, but the increase was not statistically significant. No severe bleeding occurred in any experiments. In two systems in the study group, some clots were found at autopsy around the tip of the catheter in the portal vein. No clots were found in the arterial system.

BLOOD CHEMISTRY

Serum potassium, calcium, and glucose were replaced as needed to maintain normal levels. Serum potassium levels tended to decrease due to the high volume of urine output. However, the relatively lower serum potassium levels did not appear to cause organ function abnormalities. Sodium and chloride levels remained within normal ranges during the preservation period in both groups. (Fig. 21) Serum calcium and chloride levels remained stable. (Fig. 22) Total protein ranged from 4.0-6.1 g/dL. Albumin ranged from 1.4 ± 0.1 to 3.1 ± 0.7 g/dL. (Fig. 23) Serum

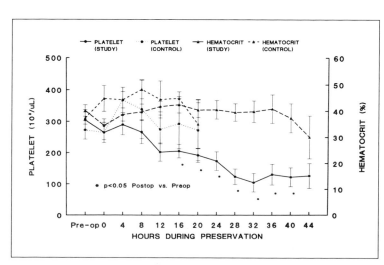

Fig. 19. Changes in platelet and hematocrit levels during preservation.

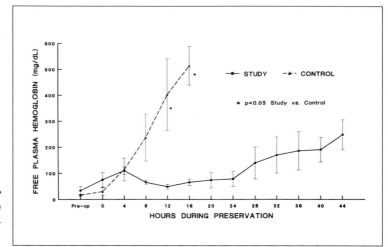

Fig. 20. Changes in free plasma hemoglobin levels in two groups during the preservation period.

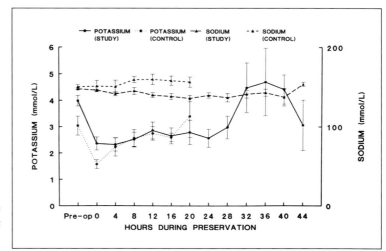

Fig. 21. Changes in serum potassium and sodium levels during preservation.

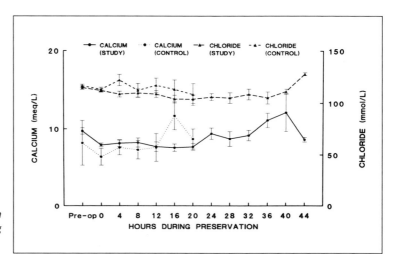

Fig. 22. Serum total calcium and chloride levels during preservation.

osmolarity ranged from 291-320 mOsm/kg. These parameters were quite stable during the preservation period. In the control group, blood chemistries were also stable.

Hormone Levels

Serum cortisol concentrations ranged from 8-60 µg/dL during the preservation period. Serum insulin levels ranged from 6-400 µU/ml during the preservation period. The higher concentration of insulin in some organ blocks resulted from the presence of insulin in the infusion solutions. The serum thyroxine (T4) concentration level was 0.9-1.7 µg/dL during the preservation period. This level was lower

than normal because the preservation block did not include the thyroid gland.

Tissue Wet/Dry Weight Ratio and Pathology Study

At the end of the experiments, the mean myocardium wet/dry weight ratio was 4.61 ± 0.23 vs. 4.59 ± 0.10 for normal dog hearts. The liver tissue wet/dry weight ratio averaged 3.64 ± 0.12 vs. 3.61 ± 0.08 for normal dog livers. The mean kidney wet/dry weight ratio was 5.54 ± 0.12 vs. 4.70 ± 0.16 for normal dogs. ($p<0.05$, Fig. 24) Lung tissue wet/dry weight ratio was 5.28 ± 0.15 at the beginning of preservation. It increased to 5.47

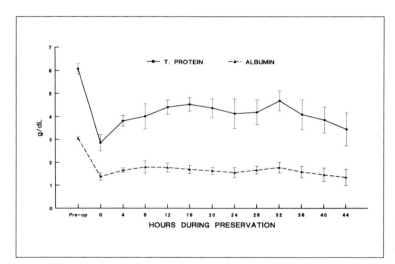

Fig. 23. Changes in serum total protein and albumin levels during preservation.

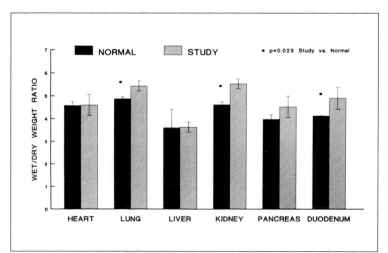

Fig. 24. Comparison in tissue wet/dry weight ratios after preservation with the ratios obtained from normal dogs.

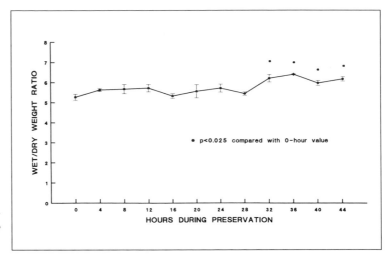

Fig. 25. Changes in lung tissue wet/dry ratios during the preservation period.

± 0.19 at 32 hours and 5.98 ± 0.12 at 40 hours. (p<0.05, Fig. 25)

CAUSES OF DEATH

In group 1A, the only cause of early death was hyperkalemia. In our experiments, 5% dextran containing no more than 0.5 g/L of potassium chloride was given intravenously. The drip was slow (1-2 ml/min). However, even with this low speed of infusion and the high volume of urine output, three systems developed ventricular fibrillation and resuscitation was unsuccessful. For the systems that survived longest, infection caused deterioration of the organs because the experiments were performed under nonsterile or semisterile conditions.

In the control group, death was primarily caused by severe liver congestion resulting in unstable circulation and premature renal failure.

TRANSPLANTATION OF THE LUNGS AFTER PRESERVATION

SELECTION OF RECIPIENT DOGS

The left lungs from the organ block in group 1B were transplanted after more than 24 hours of preservation. Preservation times were 24 hours (3 dogs), 25 hours (1 dog), 30 hours (1 dog), and 33 hours (1 dog), averaging 26.7 ±1.4 hours. The body weights of recipients and donors were matched within ± 3 kg.

TRANSPLANTATION OPERATION

The transplantation technique was a modification of that reported by Veith and Richards.[1] Each dog was anesthetized with sodium pentobarbital (30 mg/kg), intubated, and artificially ventilated. The chest was opened through the left fifth intercostal space. The left pulmonary artery was dissected free from its origin to the first branch. The pericardium was opened over the main pulmonary artery. The right main pulmonary artery was dissected free, and a 10 mm IVM OC hydraulic vascular occluder (In Vivo Metric, Healdsburg, CA) was sutured around it for later occlusion. The pericardial incision was extended inferiorly, exposing the anterior aspect of the left atrium and the left inferior pulmonary vein. The mainstem bronchus was separated from the left atrium. Two atraumatic clamps were placed across the left pulmonary artery, and the left pulmonary artery was divided distal to its first branch. The left mainstem bronchus was occluded with an angled atraumatic clamp and divided proximal to the origin of the upper lobe.

The left atrium was further mobilized by dividing the fat and visceral pericardium along its superior border. Atraumatic clamps were placed across the left atrium as far medially as possible without occluding the right pulmonary veins. The left pulmonary veins were transected at their junction with the left atrium, and the intervening tissue was incised over a clamp. The left lung was removed.

In the preservation block, heparin sodium (5 mg) was infused into the venous line. Dissection of the left lung was performed to expose the left pulmonary artery, the left mainstem bronchus, and the left atrium, as in the recipient. A 0 suture was used to encircle the left pulmonary artery. The pericardium over the main pulmonary artery was opened. A transfusion cannula was inserted into the left pulmonary artery through the main pulmonary artery, and fast infusion of cooled Collins solution was administered to cool the left lung. The suture around the left pulmonary artery was tied over the infusing cannula as close to the main pulmonary artery as possible. The left atrium was opened for fluid drainage. After 1000 ml of preservation solution had been infused and the lung tissue was cold enough, the left lung was removed. The pulmonary artery, the left mainstem bronchus, and the left atrium were cut as far away from the left lung as possible to facilitate transplantation. The removed left lung was wrapped in an ice-cooled wet towel and placed in the recipient for anastomosis.

The cut end of the recipient pulmonary artery was trimmed, and the common opening of the left pulmonary artery and its first branch was used for anastomosis. In the donor pulmonary artery, a linear incision 3-5 mm in length was made at one side of the pulmonary artery to facilitate creation of a large arterial anastomosis. Both ends of the left atrium were anastomosed using two everting mattress sutures of 4-0 prolene. Air was flushed out with saline before the sutures were tied off. Next, the bronchial anastomosis was performed. Two 3-0 prolene sutures were used for end-to-end anastomosis. After the bronchial anastomosis was completed, the bronchial clamp was removed, allowing expansion and ventilation of the transplanted left lung.

The donor and recipient pulmonary arteries were anastomosed with continuous 4-0 prolene sutures. Saline solution was used to fill the artery and expel air before the last stitch was placed. The clamps were released, and any leaks were repaired. The chest was closed in layers, and the hydraulic occluder was led out through the incision.

TREATMENT OF THE RECIPIENT ANIMALS AFTER TRANSPLANTATION

The right pulmonary artery was occluded after transplantation. In three recipients, the occlusion was performed immediately after transplantation. In the other three dogs, the occlusion was performed 0-6 hours after transplantation because of lung damage sustained during the transplantation procedure. The dogs were maintained on anesthetic and artificially ventilated after the operation. A gas mixture of 50% O_2, 3% CO_2, and 47% N_2 was used for ventilation. A Gould pressure transducer was connected to the inspiration tubing for continuous measuring of inspiratory pressures, and tidal volume was recorded during the observation period for airway resistance calculations. An arterial catheter was placed in the femoral artery for arterial pressure monitoring and blood gas sampling. A venous catheter was placed in the femoral vein for fluid infusion and blood sampling. Arterial blood samples were taken every hour for blood gas measurement, and venous blood samples were taken every four hours for hematology, blood chemistry and enzyme measurements. An intravenous drip of 5% glucose plus penicillin (1,000,000 units/L) and Flagyl (500 mg/L) was given slowly. The animal was sacrificed after 24 hours of observation, and lung tissues were examined for pathologic changes after transplantation.

HEMODYNAMIC AND FUNCTIONAL STUDIES AFTER LUNG TRANSPLANTATION

BLOOD PRESSURES

Arterial blood pressures remained stable after the transplantation without the need for blood transfusion or inotropic drug administration. Aortic systolic pressures ranged from 121 ± 2 to 141 ± 5 mmHg, aortic diastolic pressures ranged from 74 ± 2 to 91 ± 4 mmHg, and pulse pressures ranged from 47 ± 2 to 51 ± 4 mmHg. Arterial blood pressure was slightly lower during the observation period because some blood loss occurred in

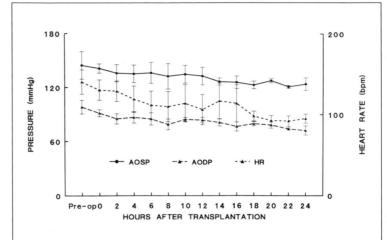

Fig. 26. Blood pressures and heart rates of the recipients after left lung transplantation. AOSP: aortic systolic pressure; AODP: aortic diastolic pressure; HR: heart rate.

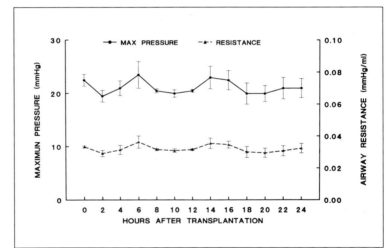

Fig. 27. Maximum respiratory pressure and airway resistance after transplantation.

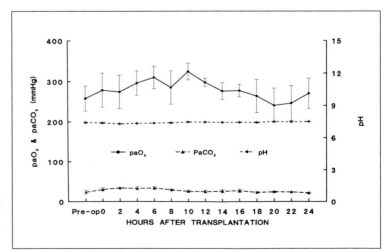

Fig. 28. Arterial oxygen tension (paO$_2$), arterial carbon dioxide tension (paCO$_2$), and pH levels after transplantation.

the chest. The heart rate ranged from 90 ± 6 to 130 ± 13 bpm. (Fig. 26) No arrhythmia occurred after transplantation. After the observation period, the heart was examined, and very few morphologic changes were found.

LUNG FUNCTION

Tidal volume ranged from 600-700 ml after transplantation. Maximum airway pressure ranged from 19 ± 1 to 24 ± 2 mmHg, and calculated airway resistance ranged from 0.029 ± 0.002 to 0.036 ± 0.002 mmHg/ml during the observation period. These values did not change appreciably after transplantation. (Fig. 27) Arterial oxygen tension was maintained from 240 ± 43 to 310 ± 28 mmHg, arterial carbon dioxide tension was maintained from 24 ± 4 to 34 ± 2 mmHg, and arterial pH was maintained from 7.33 ± 0.04 to 7.51 ± 0.02 (Fig. 28). In two transplanted lungs, where some damage was caused by longer operations, the damage spread after transplantation; some areas of atelectasis were found and frequent lung expansions were required. In one dog, oxygen tensions were low after transplantation, and opposite pulmonary artery occlusion was also delayed. This lung had some scar tissue and was hard to expand. At autopsy, heart worms were discovered in the distal pulmonary arteries. The mean lung tissue wet/dry ratio obtained 24 hours after transplantation was 5.23 ± 0.23. This ratio was higher than that of normal dog lungs (4.91 ± 0.10), but the difference was not statistically significant (p=0.18152).

FUNCTION OF OTHER RELATED ORGANS

In all liver-related enzyme studies, AST increased gradually after transplantation. However, ALT increased only slightly after 16 hours. ALP and GGT remained stable after transplantation. (Fig. 29) Total bilirubin increased from 0.1 to 0.23 mg/dL at 24 hours, but the increase was not statistically significant. Total LDH level increased twofold at 24 hours; however, the highest value was still within normal range. The LDH_1 isoenzyme level increased during the observation period but remained within the normal range. Both LDH_3 and LDH_5 isoenzyme levels remained normal or slightly below normal during the observation period. (Fig. 30) The CK levels increased dramatically after transplantation as a reaction to surgery. The CK-MB level also increased after transplantation. (Fig. 31) Serum amylase levels remained stable after transplantation, as did serum lactic acid levels. Serum potassium, sodium, chloride and calcium levels remained normal during the observation period. Serum protein and albumin levels were slightly lower after transplantation because no blood transfusions were given.

Red blood cell levels were stable after transplantation. White blood cell levels increased during the observation period; this

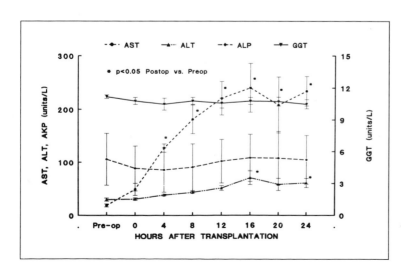

Fig. 29. Changes in serum aspartate amino-transferase (AST), serum alanine aminotransferase (ALT), serum alkaline phosphatase (ALP), and gamma glutamyl transpeptidase (GGT) levels after left lung transplantation.

increase probably resulted from bacterial contamination or from a reaction to surgery. Platelet levels were stable after transplantation.

All recipient dogs maintained normal urine output after transplantation. Tests indicated good renal function, including stable or lower blood urea nitrogen and creatinine levels.

DISCUSSION

A major problem with using dogs for autoperfusion organ preservation studies is severe liver congestion. This congestion is thought to be caused by hepatic vein sphincter constriction.[2,3] Such sphincters are known to be present in several animal species, such as rabbits, cats, and monkeys, but the most

prominent are in dogs. There is some evidence of their presence in humans.[4-7] Liver congestion usually persists throughout the experiment. The congestion reduces venous inflow and effective circulating volume, causing early deterioration of the whole system. The need for inotropic drug infusion was reported in similar studies.[8,9] In our previous studies, inotropic drug administration was not required. However, the preservation blocks were usually jeopardized if severe liver congestion occurred. A similar phenomenon was seen in the control group in this study. For this preservation system, liver congestion was a bottle-neck for all the preserved organs. One dramatic result of using HIT was the

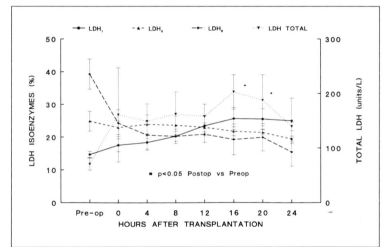

Fig. 30. Changes in the levels of serum lactic dehydrogenase (LDH) and its isoenzymes 1, 3 and 5 after left lung transplantation.

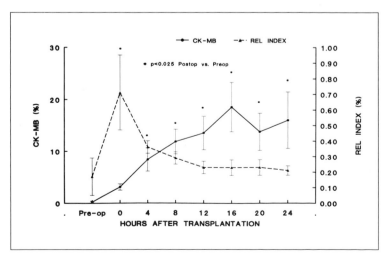

Fig. 31. Changes in total serum creatine phosphokinase (CK) and CK-MB after transplantation.

reduction or elimination of liver congestion. When there was no liver congestion, the entire organ system functioned extremely well. Hemodynamic stability was easily maintained by slow blood transfusion, and no additional interventions were required.

The heart was very well preserved. Maintenance of normal heart function was demonstrated by stable pressures, heart rate, left ventricular maximum dp/dt, and lack of arrhythmias. Within 36 hours, the heart was not enlarged, the color was normal and no pericardial effusion was seen. Although the pericardium was not opened in any of the experiments, no excess fluid was found in the pericardium even at the end of the experiment. This was in contrast to previous heart-lung autoperfusion preparations in which the pericardium had to be opened after 8-12 hours due to excess fluid.[10] At the end of the experiment, myocardial wet/dry weight ratio was only slightly higher than that found in normal dog hearts. Cardiac output was in the range of 400-550 ml/min. This was related to the small mass of the organ block. Systemic resistance remained stable within 24-36 hours of preservation but tended to increase after 36 hours.

An unusual finding in this study was the high sensitivity of the heart to hyperkalemia. Three deaths occurred before 48 hours, and all were related to hyperkalemia, even when the myocardium appeared to be in an excellent functional state. Dextrose or Ringer's solution was routinely used to replace volume loss during organ harvesting. Urine output was usually high during the preservation period, especially at the beginning of preservation. High urine production resulted in overall hypokalemia, and intravenous dripping of potassium chloride was usually required to replace potassium loss. Due to the relatively small blood volume of the system, fluctuation of serum potassium occurred more easily than in the normal animal. In three experiments, when early deaths occurred, the actual potassium levels were approximately 6-7 mMol/L, which was well tolerated in other studies in which HIT was not used. On the other hand, relatively lower serum potassium levels were well tolerated by the system. In

most experiments, serum potassium levels were approximately 2.0-2.5 mMol/L during the preservation period, and arrhythmia occasionally occurred when serum potassium levels fell below 2.0 mMol/L. Extreme care was exercised in administering potassium. We usually used a separate solution for potassium administration, and the concentration of potassium was kept below 0.05%. Double regulators were applied to prevent an accidental fast flush, and serum potassium levels were checked every two hours. If potassium-containing penicillin is used, such as penicillin G potassium, the separate potassium infusion is omitted. In our limited experience, a relatively lower serum potassium level poses less risk than higher potassium levels in the autoperfusion preparation using HIT.

Preservation of the lungs has been investigated extensively since the late 1960s. Progress has been slow, and consistent clinical results have not been achieved when preservation times exceed six hours.[11-13] For several reasons, preserving lung tissue is much more difficult than preserving other organs. First, the unique, delicate architecture of the lung poses a special problem in preservation. Methods effective for the short-term storage of kidneys, livers, and hearts do not necessarily work for lungs. Second, total functional dependence is placed on the preserved lung after it is transplanted, making evaluation of functional adequacy more critical during preservation.[14-17] Several techniques have been used for lung preservation, including single-flush hypothermia, mechanical perfusion, in situ donor core-cooling and autoperfusion. However, preservation times are still too short, and the results are unpredictable. A significant problem associated with these techniques is that excessive water and metabolic wastes produced during the preservation period accumulate in the lung, damaging its tissue and finally causing premature pulmonary edema.[18-20]

The preservation of the lungs in this study has been very impressive. In group 1A, lung function was well maintained for up to 44 hours. No pulmonary edema was noted before 40 hours. However, lung color changes occurred earlier than functional changes. The earliest change occurred at 20 hours, and the latest change started at 36 hours. These changes were mainly related to lung protection during harvesting. Surface damage caused by drying out during harvesting was a major cause of lung damage. Red spots and local atelectasis could be found after 40 hours of preservation. Any laceration of lung tissue during harvesting will cause bleeding and air leaks after the organ block is placed in the water bath. However, if the surface of the lungs is well protected by moisturized towels during harvesting and preservation, good lung function will be maintained well beyond 36 hours.

Protecting the lungs during preservation is also very important. Because the lungs float in the bath solution, their surface must be covered by moisturized towels. In our experiments, we not only covered the lungs but also covered the bath tank with a sterile plastic sheet. In this way, all the organs were protected from drying out and contamination.

After the lungs are removed from the chest cage, negative pressure ceases to exist, and the lungs tend to collapse. If a lobe is allowed to remain collapsed for an extended period of time, atelectasis will follow. Using PEEP during preservation helps to maintain satisfactory lung expansion. However, frequent observation of the lungs is required so that any collapsed portion can be reexpanded.

In this study, hemolysis caused by untyped blood was found in four experiments in both groups as evidenced by sudden increases in free plasma hemoglobin levels. Severe hemolysis could also accelerate early lung color changes.

Lung tissue wet/dry weight ratios exhibited only a small increase at the end of 40 hours; this increase was not statistically different from the ratios of normal dog lungs. In group 1B, the left lungs were transplanted after more than 24 hours of preservation; lung function was excellent after transplantation. Those lungs were usually in very good condition after more than 24 hours of preservation; no evidence of lung damage was visible. In most lungs, even the surface color change was minimal. Sometimes the left lung showed some damage after transplantation, mainly induced by longer anastomosis times. When

this occurred, delayed opposite pulmonary artery occlusion was performed. However, surface damage also persisted after transplantation. The longest preservation time before transplantation in this group was 33 hours. We have not seen any other report in which the lung could be preserved for such a long period of time and then transplanted with concomitant opposite pulmonary artery ligation.

The effect of HIT on liver preservation was dramatic. When HIT is not used, liver congestion may begin as soon as the abdomen is opened. Liver function deterioration then occurs progressively during the preservation period and may cause hemodynamic instability. However, in the study group, liver congestion was minimal or absent during operation. Liver congestion sometimes occurred during the preservation period, but an intravenous injection of HIT eliminated congestion and quickly restored normal function. Liver-related enzyme levels increased immediately after the operation, then decreased during the preservation period. We believe the early increase in liver-related enzyme levels was mainly caused by surgical manipulation, including damage to skeletal muscles and other organs. The increase of liver-related enzyme levels was not uniform, and the levels remained unchanged or increased very little in most systems. However, the enzyme levels increased dramatically in a few experiments despite the use of HIT. We cannot explain the discrepancies in these changes. One possible explanation may be that, when we obtained the plasma from hibernating animals, their depth of hibernation was not uniform, which may have affected the concentration of HIT in the plasma. This speculation can only be substantiated when the full biochemical characterization of HIT is completed. In the control group, liver congestion was always present, and sometimes it was severe enough to cause an unstable circulation. The increases of liver-related enzymes, including AST, ALT, LDH and ALP, were noted much earlier and were more severe in the control group, suggesting that liver damage occurred much earlier in the absence of HIT.

Extensive dissection is always necessary to remove all the organs. We imagined that massive blood transfusion might be required after surgery. To our surprise, bleeding was usually minimal, in contrast to the earlier heart-lung autoperfusion preparation in which bleeding was a severe problem.[21] We believe that this low occurrence of bleeding is related to the production of clotting factors by the functional liver. If excess transfusion is required to maintain satisfactory blood pressure, bleeding points usually exist in the system. Common bleeding sites include loose ties or staples at the stumps of the intercostal arteries and lacerations of the liver. Bleeding points on the descending aorta, heart, pancreas, and kidneys are very easy to find. The most unnoticeable bleeders are usually from small lacerations of the liver. If unexplained excessive blood loss occurs, a thorough inspection of the liver is indicated. In several experiments, small numbers of clots were found around the catheters in the portal vein, which might be related to a slow flow rate in the portal vein and the high coagulability level of the blood of dogs. A small amount of heparin in the infusion solution would probably help prevent clot formation in this model.

We believe that the kidneys contributed significantly to organ survival in the system. In all other studies in which only the heart and lungs are used, accumulation of water and metabolic wastes always causes deterioration of the entire system. Good renal function appears to be important in long-term organ preservation, because the removal of excess water and metabolic wastes is vital for tissue protection.[22] No premature renal failure occurred in the study group, and no unusual tissue edema occurred during the preservation period. Laboratory tests for BUN and creatinine indicated good renal function during the preservation period. In contrast to the heart-lung autoperfusion preparation without the kidneys, good renal function kept our system in a relatively normal state and eliminated the need for sophisticated hemodialysis or cross-circulation.[21,23,24]

Hemolysis has always been another major problem in heart-lung autoperfusion preparations.[24] The damage appears to be caused when the blood elements pass through plastic tubing. In the study group, free plasma hemoglobin levels had increased only twofold at 24 hours. The low incidence of hemolysis was probably related to the fact that blood perfused a natural vasculature; no foreign materials were involved. Another factor may have been the protective effects of HIT on erythrocytes. The increase of free plasma hemoglobin levels in the control group was not uniform. Severe increases in free plasma hemoglobin occurred in only two experiments. Sudden increases in free plasma hemoglobin levels occurred after blood transfusion. Similar increases occurred twice in group 1A, although the increases were not as severe as those in the control group. In all those experiments in which free plasma hemoglobin levels increased, the levels usually decreased within 6-8 hours after the initial increase. The changes appeared to be related more to the transfusion of untyped blood than to blood damage within the system.

In hematological studies, one consistent finding in our experiments was the progressive decrease in white blood cell and platelet counts during the course of preservation. The decrease was severe and persistent, and the reduction worsened as preservation continued. There are several possible reason for the reduction. First, there is no bone marrow, which can maintain a continuous blood cell supply. Second, contamination of the system also consumes white blood cells. Third, aggregation and sequestration of white blood cells in lung tissue also play a role in this change. In pathologic studies, serial lung sections showed clumps of white blood cells in the vascular space. These findings suggested the possibility that one reason for final organ dysfunction during the autoperfusion studies might be embolization from platelet and neutrophil aggregates in the heart, lungs, liver and kidneys. Spontaneous contrast is associated with circulating platelet and platelet-neutrophil aggregates. Our previous clinical studies showed that platelet aggregates appeared with myocardial infarction and persisted for several days.[25] In the canine model, the occurrence of circulating platelet and neutrophil aggregates can be detected by ultrasound.[26] Certain drugs such as epinephrine could increase the number of these aggregates. In previous studies, ultrasonic detection of large numbers of particles in perfusates during cardiac surgery, as a result of cardiopulmonary bypass, was associated with multiorgan failure and a poor prognosis.[25,26] Echocardiographic examinations were performed when the organ block was preserved. The inferior vena cava contained particles that moved with the blood flow and appeared to increase in size and number during the course of the autoperfusion study. Unstable hemodynamics and early deaths occurred in the organ blocks with the most aggregates. The significance of platelet aggregation in relation to tissue damage is still controversial, and this issue is under further investigation.

Hormonal assays for both cortisol and insulin in the preservation block were normal or higher than normal, due to supplementation of these factors in the infusion solution. The pancreas is included in the preservation block, the infusion of insulin may not be required. Because the thyroid was not included, thyroxine level was always low in the preservation block. The beneficial effect of adding thyroxine to the infusion solution still needs further study.

Hibernation is a biological phenomenon in which a number of unique physiological changes occur, including hypothermia, bradycardia, long-term hypophagia, and generalized metabolic depression. In naturally hibernating ground squirrels, body temperature is lowered to just above ambient levels (as low as 0°C), heart rate decreases from approximately 400 bpm to as low as 2 bpm, and respiratory rate slows from approximately 200 bpm to as low as 1 bpm.[27] Very little is known about the specific biochemical mechanisms involved in the initiation of hibernation.[28,29] Dawe and Spurrier[30] first presented evidence for the presence of a hibernation factor in the blood of the hibernating woodchuck and ground squirrel. This factor was designated as the hibernation induction trigger (HIT).[31-33] Previous studies have shown that HIT in winter-hibernating animals could induce hibernation in summer-active hibernators placed in a cold room. The "trigger" was not found in the blood of summer-active hibernators.[30] The hibernation induction trigger is extracted from deeply hibernating animals (woodchuck, ground squirrel, brown cave bat, and black bear). Debate about the existence of HIT has persisted since early attempts to chemically characterize the substance were inconclusive.[33] However, the biological effects of HIT have been demonstrated in many studies. HIT has been utilized to induce hibernation in mammals.[34-36] Infusion of a hibernation induction trigger into a non-hibernating primate (*Macacca mulatta*) induced profound behavioral and physiologic depression, including hypothermia, bradycardia, long-term hypophagia without significant weight loss, an anesthetized state and decreased renal function[31,32,37] as described in Chapter 1. Kidneys from hibernating animals have been kept viable for up to 10 days.[38] Previous studies have also shown that the erythrocytes in hibernating animals demonstrate increased resistance in osmotic fragility tests and often appear to be "folded-over" in cold blood drawn during hibernation. In Spurrier and Dawe's study,[27] when red cells were incubated at 5°, 20° and 37°C for several hours in the plasma, approximately 40%-50% of the ground squirrel's cells were folded in the hibernator's serum at 5°C, but when the cells were warmed to 37°C they unfolded. Unfolded cells did not refold by simple application of cold. Human red cells did not fold over, nor did the erythrocytes from active ground squirrels. Neither human cells nor ground squirrel cells agglutinated in ground squirrel serum at low temperatures.[27] Studies of blood and circulatory changes in hibernating animals have also found that in hibernation erythrocytes have an increased resistance to hemolysis and higher levels of unsaturated fatty acids.[27] Also, HIT has been shown to cause a significant change in renal function and creatinine clearance.[31] HIT has been hypothesized to be nonspecies specific, because it reacts with receptor sites in the brains of monkeys to suppress physiologic processes. The opiate antagonists, naloxone or naltrexone, either reversed or retarded these alterations[32] as detailed in Chapter 1.

We believe that this is the first time that the beneficial effects of HIT in organ preservation have been clearly shown. However, extensive studies are needed to explore the mechanism of HIT's effect on organ survival. The reduction or elimination of liver congestion is probably related directly to the relaxation of the hepatic vein mechanism by HIT. The vasodilator effect of HIT was shown before preservation, because systemic blood pressure reduced to half when HIT-containing plasma was injected intravenously in dogs. Previous studies have demonstrated that the intravenous injection into dogs of a number of substances caused a marked engorgement of the liver, whether in vivo or in vitro. In an intact animal, hepatic congestion was accompanied by severe shock, as evidenced by an extreme decrease in arterial blood pressure and death of the animal if the dose of the substance was sufficiently large.[39] The specific anatomic location of the constriction is not totally clear. However, several mechanisms control the outflow of blood from the portal vein bed and liver, including contractile hepatic veins, contractile sublobular veins, Deysach "small sluice channel" and sinusoid outlet sphincters.[4,6] In laboratory studies using dogs, local administration of large doses of epinephrine (0.5 ml for dogs weighing 8 to 25 kg) prior to the injection of the contrast medium completely prevented contraction of the hepatic vein sphincters. However, the same dose of epinephrine given after the sphincter mechanisms were set in operation failed to release the already contracted sphincters.[40] In this study, we found that, even when the hepatic vein was contracted, injection of HIT-containing plasma could easily release the contraction. The potent vasodilator effect of HIT and the differences in its reaction from that of epinephrine suggest that extensive study is needed to identify the mechanism of this benefit.

It appears that the effect of HIT on extending organ survival time was not limited to its vasodilator mechanism in this study. In the control group in which HIT was not used, lung deterioration began earlier than in the study group. Since hibernating animals have very low metabolic rates, it is possible that HIT may also reduce metabolism or improve membrane stability in living tissue. Evidence from our other study has suggested

this possibility. We will discuss this issue in Chapter 6. Based on our preliminary experiments, the beneficial effects of HIT on autoperfusion multiorgan preservation have been clearly demonstrated in several organs. The possible mechanisms involved might be related to the following effects of HIT: 1) inhibition of tissue metabolism, 2) reduction or elimination of liver congestion, and 3) reduction of hemolysis.

One limitation in this study was that all experiments were performed under semisterile conditions. Bacterial contamination usually occurred during the operation or the preservation period. Gross infection, when it occurred, resulted in rapid deterioration and death. A totally sterile procedure should result in increased survival times.[41]

References

1. Veith FJ, Richards K: Improved technique for canine lung transplantation. Ann Surg 1970; 171:553-558.

2. Chien S, Todd EP, Diana JN, O'Connor WN: A simple technique for multiorgan preservation. J Thorac Cardiovasc Surg 1988; 95:55-61.

3. Calne RY: Preservation of the liver. In: Calne RY, ed. Liver Transplantation. New York: Grune & Stratton, 1983:17-23.

4. Knisely MH, Harding F, Debacker H: Hepatic sphincters. Science 1957; 125:1023-1026.

5. Gibson JB: The hepatic veins in man and their sphincter mechanisms. J Anat Lond 1959; 93:369-379.

6. Walker WF, Macdonald JS, Pickard C: Hepatic vein sphincter mechanism in the dog. Brit J surg 1960; 48:218-220.

7. Andrews WHH, Hecker R, Maegraith BG: The actyion of adrenaline, noradrenaline, acetylcholine and histamine on the perfused liver of the monkey, cat and rabbit. J Physiol (London) 1956; 132:509-521.

8. Prieto M, Baron P, Andreone PA, et al: Multiple ex vivo organ preservation with warm whole blood. J Heart Transplant 1988; 7:227-237.

9. Prieto M, Androne PA, Baron P et al: Multiple organ retrieval and preservation with normothermic autoperfusion. Transplant Proc

1988; 20:827-828.

10. Robicsek F, Pruitt JR, Sanger PW, Daugherty HK, Moore M, Bagby E: The maintenance of function of the donor heart in the extracorporeal stage and during transplantation. Ann Thorac Surg 1968; 6:330-342.

11. Haverich A, Scott WC, Jamieson SW: Twenty years of lung preservation-a review. Heart Transplant 1985; 4:234-240.

12. Puskas JD, Cardoso PFG, Mayer E, Shi S, Slutsky AS, Patterson GA: Equivalent eighteen-hour lung preservation with low-potassium dextran or Euro-Collins solution after prostaglandin E-1 infusion. J Thorac Cardiovasc Surg 1992; 104:83-89.

13. Schueler S, De Valeria PA, Hatanaka M, et al: Successful 24-hour lung preservation with donor core cooling and leukocyte depletion in an orthotopic double lung transplantation model. J Thorac Cardiovasc Surg 1992; 104:73-82.

14. Modry DL, Jirsch DW, Boehme G, Overton T, Fisk RL, Couves CM: Hypothermic perfusion preservation of the isolated dog lung. Ann Thorac Surg 1973; 16:583-597.

15. Crane R, Torres M, Hagstrom JWC, Koerner SK, Veith FJ: Twenty-four-hour preservation and transplantation of the lung without functional impairment. Surg Forum 1975; 26:111-113.

16. Veith FJ, Montefusco CM: Lung preservation. In: Toledo-Pereyra LH, ed. Basic Concepts of Organ Procurement, Perfusion, and Preservation for Transplantation. New York: Academic Press, 1982:279-299.

17. Montefusco CM, Veith FJ: Lung transplantation. In: Flye MW, ed. Principles of Organ Transplantation. Philadelphia: W.B.Saunders Co., 1989:413-435.

18. Schueler S, Warnecke H, Hetzer R, Loitz F, Topalidis T, Borst HG: The limits of cold ischemia for preservation of the lung. J Heart Transplant 1984; 4:70-75.

19. Mancini MC, Griffith BP, Borovetz HS, Hardesty RL: Static lung preservation. Curr Surg 1985; 42:23-25.

20. Locke TJ, Hooper TL, Flecknell PA, McGregor CGA: Preservation of the lung: comparison of topical cooling and cold crystalloid pulmonary perfusion. J Thorac Cardiovasc Surg 1988; 96:789-795.

21. Stewart RW, Morimoto T, Golding LR, Harasaki H, Olsen E, Nose Y: Canine heart-lung autoperfusion. Trans Am Soc Artif Int Organs 1985; 31:206-210.

22. Chien S, Diana JN, Todd EP, O'Connor WN, Marion T, Smith K: New autoperfusion preparation for long-term organ preservation. Circulation 1988; 78 (Suppl. III):58-65.

23. Tam W, Robicsek F, Daugherty HK, Mullen DC: Autoperfusing heart-lung preparation: prolonged survival by extracorporeal symbiosis. Transplant Proc 1971; 3:640-642.

24. Yamada T, Bosher LH, Richardson GM: Observations on the autoperfusing heart-lung preparation. Trans Am Soc Artif Int Organs 1965; 11:192-196.

25. Mahony C, Sublett KL, Harrison MR: Resolution of spontaneous contrast with platelet disaggregatory therapy (trifluoperazine). Am J Cardiol 1989; 63:1009-1010.

26. Mahony C, Spain MG: Association of platelet and neutrophil aggregates with spontaneous contrast by echocardiography in dogs. Circulation 1986; 74 (Suppl. II):144-144. (Abstract)

27. Spurrier WA, Dawe AR: Several blood and circulatory changes in the hibernation of the 13-lined ground squirrel, *Citellus tridecemlineatus*. Comp Biochem Physiol 1973; 44A:267-282.

28. Oeltgen PR, Bergmann LC, Spurrier WA, Jones SB: Isolation of a hibernation inducing trigger(s) from the plasma of hibernating woodchucks. Prep Biochem 1978; 8:171-188.

29. Oeltgen PR, Spurrier WA, Bergmann LC: Hemoglobin alterations of the 13-lined ground squirrel while in various activity states. Comp Biochem Physiol 1979; 64B:207-211.

30. Dawe AR, Spurrier WA: Hibernation induced in ground squirrels by blood transfusions. Science 1969; 163:298-299.

31. Oeltgen PR, Blouin RA, Spurrier WA, Myers RD: Hibernation "trigger" alters renal function in the primate. Physiol Behav 1985; 34:79-81.

32. Oeltgen PR, Walsh JW, Hamann SR, Randall DC, Spurrier WA, Myers RD: Hibernation "trigger": opioid-like inhibitory action on brain function of the monkey. Pharmacol Biochem Behav 1982; 17:1271-1274.

33. Bigelow WG: Intellectual humility in medical practice and research. Surgery 1969; 65: 1-9.

34. Castaneda AR, Arnar O, Schmidt-Habelman P, Moller JH, Zamora R: Cardiopulmonary autotransplantation in primates. J Cardiovasc Surg 1972; 13:523-531.

35. Bruce DS, Tuggy ML, Pearson PJ: Summer hibernation induced in ground squirrels (*Citellus tridecemlineatus*) by urine and plasma from hibernating bats (*Myotis lucifugus* or *Eptesicus fuscus*). Cryobiology 1984; 21:371-374.

36. Ruit KA, Bruce DS, Chien PP, Oeltgen PR, Wellborn JR, Nilekani SP: Summer hibernation in ground squirrels (*Citellus tridecemlineatus*) induced by injection of whole or fractionated plasma from hibernating black bears (*Ursus americanus*). J Therm Biol 1987; 12:135-138.

37. Myers RD, Oeltgen PR, Spurrier WA: Hibernation "trigger" injected in brain induces hypothermia and hypophagia in the monkey. Brain Res Bull 1981; 7:691-695.

38. Green CJ, Fuller BJ, Ross B, Marriott S, Simpkin S: Storage of organs from ground-squirrels during and after hibernation. The 20th Annual Meeting for The Society for Cryobiology 1983; 149-149. (Abstract)

39. Thomas WD, Essex HE: Observations on the hepatic venous circulation with special reference to the sphincteric mechanism. Am J Physiol 1949; 158:303-310.

40. Moreno AH, Rousselot LM, Burchell AR, Bono RF, Burke JH: Studies on the outflow tracts of the liver: II. On the outflow tracts of the canine liver with particular reference to its regulation by the hepatic vein sphincter mechanisms. Ann Surg 1962; 155:427-433.

41. Robicsek F, Masters TN, Duncan GD, Denyer MH, Rise HE, Etchison M: An autoperfused heart-lung-preparation: Metabolism and function. Heart Transplant 1985; 4:334-338.

CHAPTER 5

EXTENDING ORGAN SURVIVAL TIME USING DELTA OPIOID (DADLE)

In Chapter 4, we reported that infusion of plasma from hibernating woodchucks into the multiorgan preservation block extended tissue survival time significantly. Previous studies have also shown that a *delta* opioid (D-Ala^2-Leu^5-Enkephalin, DADLE) can induce a hibernation-like state when injected into hibernators.[1,2] These findings led us to believe that infusion of DADLE would also extend tissue survival time. This chapter presents the experimental results of using a *delta* opioid (DADLE) to extend effective tissue survival time in the multiorgan preservation block.

MATERIAL AND METHODS

ANIMALS STUDIED
Six adult mongrel dogs of either sex weighing 17-30 kg each were used in this study. DADLE was given before and after the operation. To obtain normal organ wet/dry weight ratios, tissue samples from the heart, lungs, liver, pancreas, duodenum, and kidney were taken from ten normal dogs and used for comparison.

PRETREATMENT
All dogs were given neomycin (2 gm) orally once a day for three days before the operation to sterilize their digestive systems. The dogs were fasted for five hours before the operation. DADLE (25 mg) was injected intravenously two hours before surgery. Another dose of DADLE (25 mg) was given one hour prior to the operation.

SURGICAL TECHNIQUE
The procedure used to harvest the organs was the same as that described in Chapter 3.

Interventions

The temperature was maintained at approximately 32°C by heating the water bath with a constant temperature circulator. Artificial respiration was maintained with a Harvard volume-cycled respirator at a tidal volume of 500-700 ml, a rate of 10-20 rpm, and PEEP of 2-6 cm H_2O. A gas mixture of 50% O_2 + 3% CO_2 + 47% N_2 was utilized. The following solution was given at 10-20 ml/hour through the portal vein:

    Dextrose 5%
    Calcium chloride 1 gm/L
    Insulin 50 units/L
    Mannitol 12.5 g/L
    Methylprednisolone 500 mg/L
    Penicillin 1,000,000 units/L
    Flagyl 500 mg/L

Another 5% dextrose solution containing potassium (0.5 g/L) was infused slowly through the portal vein to maintain serum potassium at a normal level.

A fat emulsion (Soyacal, 2 ml) and prednisolone (30 mg) were given through the portal vein every 2 hours. Blood transfusions were given to maintain aortic systolic pressure at 75-100 mmHg and CVP at 0-10 mmHg. Plasma was given instead of whole blood if the hematocrit was higher than 45%.

Application of DADLE

DADLE (7.5 mg), diluted in 2 ml of normal saline, was given through the portal vein immediately after the operation and every two hours during the preservation period. This represented a dosage of approximately 1 mg/kg, which is typically used in studies with purified opioids.

Monitoring

Aortic pressure, left ventricular pressure, left ventricular dp/dt, central venous pressure, portal venous pressure, and aortic blood flow were monitored and recorded on a SensorMedics R612 Dynograph Recorder throughout the preservation period. Temperature, urine output, bile production, and duodenal and pancreatic secretions were collected and recorded every hour. Visual changes including color, size and bleeding for each organ and respiratory pressure, tidal volume and PEEP for the lungs were recorded every hour. Arterial blood gas and hematocrit measurements were taken before the operation and every hour thereafter. Blood samples were taken before the operation and every four hours during the preservation period and used for blood chemistries, hematology, lactic acid, and enzyme measurements for heart, liver, pancreas and kidney function tests. Tissue samples were taken from the lungs every eight hours for tissue wet/dry weight ratios and electron microscope studies. At the termination of the study, specimens were taken from each organ for wet/dry weight ratios and pathologic examinations.

Determination of Tissue Wet/Dry Weight Ratios

Tissue samples used for wet/dry weight measurement were blotted to remove excess fluid, and wet weight was measured. The dry weight was determined after the samples had been in an oven at 85°C for 72 hours.

Statistical Analysis

All the laboratory tests obtained before the operation (blood gases, hematocrit, blood chemistries, hematology, lactic acid and enzymes for heart, liver, pancreas and kidney functions) were used as normal controls that were compared with the parameters obtained during the preservation period. Heart rate, blood pressures, left ventricular dp/dt, blood gases, and urine output were measured immediately after harvesting and compared with measurements obtained during the preservation period. Tissue wet/dry weight ratios for all organs were compared with those obtained from normal control dogs.

ANOVA and Student-Newman-Keuls tests were used to compare the parameters measured during the preservation period with those obtained preoperatively or immediately postoperatively. The level of significance was 0.05.

Results

The survival times of the organs ranged from 41-60 hours with a mean of 46.7 hours.

(Fig. 1) The experiments were performed under semisterile or nonsterile conditions, and infection eventually caused death in all experiments.

CARDIAC FUNCTION

Aortic systolic pressure (AOSP) remained stable throughout the experiments. AOSP ranged from 62 ± 7 mmHg to 79 ± 3 mmHg and was easily adjusted by blood or plasma infusion. No inotropic drugs were necessary. Aortic diastolic pressure ranged from 33 ± 4 to 49 ± 7 mmHg. Aortic pulse pressure ranged from 22 ± 3 to 34 ± 11 mmHg and did not fluctuate appreciably during the preservation period. (Immediately after the operation it was 28 ± 5 mmHg, and at 44 hours it was 33

± 24 mmHg.) CVP ranged from 4.9 ± 0.6 to 9.2 ± 2.9 mmHg. It increased slightly after 32 hours, but the increase was not statistically significant. The heart rate ranged from 86 ± 8 to 100 ± 12 beats per minute. It was lower than that in normal animals. (Fig. 2) Left ventricular maximum dp/dt was 1280 ± 215 mmHg/second at the beginning of preservation. It increased to 1920 ± 164 at 4 hours but decreased gradually during preservation. It was 1250 ± 353 mmHg/second at 44 hours. Left ventricular maximum dp/dt/p was 17.18 ± 2.24 (second^{-1}) at the beginning of preservation. It increased to 24.3 ± 1.8 (second^{-1}) at 4 hours and was maintained at approximately this level during the preservation period.

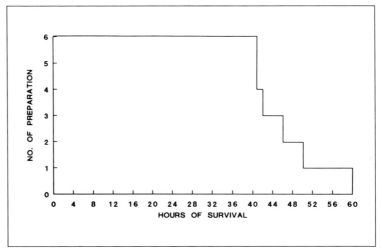

Fig. 1. Distribution of survival time in the study.

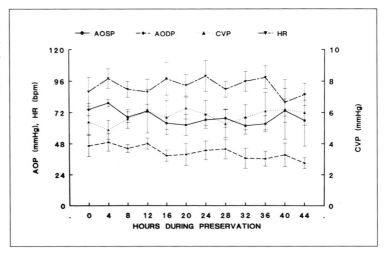

Fig. 2. Change of heart function during the preservation period. HR: heart rate; AOSP: Aortic systolic pressure; AODP: Aortic diastolic pressure; CVP: Central venous pressure.

It decreased gradually after 36 hours and was 18.99 ± 0.17 (second⁻¹) at 44 hours. (Fig. 3)

The heart remained in good condition during the preservation period. The size usually did not change within 36 hours. The pericardium was not opened in any of the experiments. No fluid was found in the pericardium at the end of the experiments. Arrhythmia occurred occasionally during preservation when serum potassium levels fell below 2 mMol/L. If severe infection occurred, the heart deteriorated before overall organ failure occurred. As was true in the HIT study, the heart was sensitive to hyperkalemia after treatment with DADLE. The heart became hypokinetic if serum potassium levels rose above normal. Lower serum potassium levels were preferred in the experiments when DADLE was used.

After preservation, the myocardium wet/dry weight ratio was 4.579 ± 0.180, which was not different from that of a normal dog heart (4.552 ± 0.127). The serum lactic acid level was 3.6 mMol/L before surgery. It increased to 7.4 mMol/L after surgery but decreased to 4.3 mMol/L at 4 hours and remained near this level during preservation. It increased to 7.8 mMol/L at 40 hours. ($p<0.05$, Fig. 4)

LUNG FUNCTION

A gas mixture of 50% O_2 + 3% CO_2 + 47% N_2 was used during the preservation

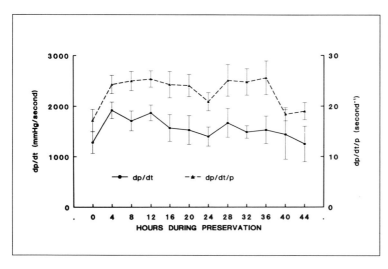

Fig. 3. Changes of left ventricular dp/dt and dp/dt/p during the preservation period.

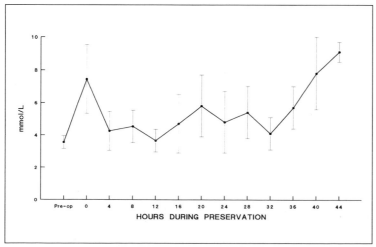

Fig. 4. Blood lactic acid levels during preservation period.

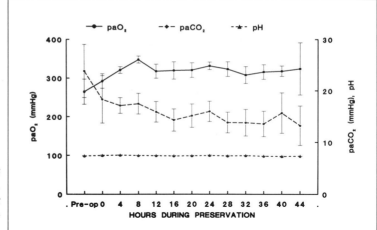

Fig. 5. Change of blood gas
values during preservation.
paO_2: Arterial oxygen tension;
$paCO_2$: Arterial carbon dioxide tension.

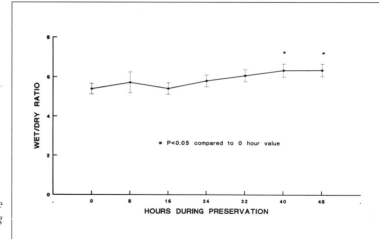

Fig. 6. Change of lung tissue
wet/dry weight ratios during
preservation.

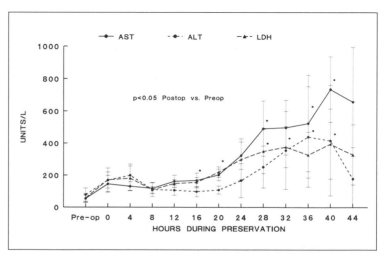

Fig. 7. Changes of blood enzymes during preservation.
AST: Aspartate amino-transferase; ALT: Alanine amino-
transferase; LDH: Lactate dehydrogenase; CK: creatinine
kinase; ALP: Alkaline phosphatase.

period. Arterial oxygen tension (paO_2) was 292 ± 18 mmHg after the organ block was placed in the bath solution. It increased to 348 ± 9 mmHg at eight hours (p<0.05) and remained near this level during preservation. It was 324 ± 67 mmHg at 44 hours. Arterial carbon dioxide tension ($paCO_2$) was 18.4 ± 4.6 mmHg at the beginning of preservation. It ranged from 13.3 ± 3.8 to 17.5 ± 2.1 mmHg during the preservation period. Arterial pH value was 7.48 ± 0.1 after surgery. It ranged from 7.29 ± 0.07 to 7.54 ± 0.06 during the preservation period and did not shift significantly. (Fig. 5) The lungs maintained good function for more than 36 hours. Lung color changes were apparent earlier than functional changes. However, the change of lung color primarily resulted from exposure of lung surfaces to air during harvesting. Lung tissue samples were obtained every eight hours for wet/dry weight ratio measurements and pathologic studies. Lung tissue wet/dry weight ratio was 5.40 ± 0.27 at the beginning of preservation. It changed to 5.81 ± 0.30 at 24 hours and increased to 6.35 ± 0.33 at 40 hours. (Fig. 6)

Liver Function

Total bile output ranged from 122-300 ml with an average of 2.7-6.1 ml/hour during the preservation period. The livers exhibited minimal changes during the preservation period. In some experiments, they showed signs of congestion, including patchy darkening and stiffness to touch during harvesting or preservation. However, they gradually returned to normal after DADLE administration. Serum AST level was 54 ± 22 U/L before surgery. It increased to 145 ± 52 U/L immediately after harvesting but decreased within 4-8 hours. It then increased gradually during preservation and reached 656 ± 353 U/L at 44 hours. The serum ALT level was 78 ± 41 U/L before surgery. It increased to 198 ± 90 U/L after surgery but decreased within 8 hours. It increased gradually after 24 hours and reached 416 ± 343 U/L at 40 hours. The increase of ALT was not equal in every experiment. In this group of animals, in only one organ block did ALT increase substantially, to 1305 U/L at 40 hours. In the other five experiments, the AST levels were all below 200 U/L. Serum LDH was 57 ± 28 U/L before surgery. It increased to 170 ± 73 after harvesting but decreased within eight hours. It increased gradually during preservation and reached 329 ± 187 U/L at 44 hours. Again, the increase of LDH was not equal. In only one experiment did the LDH level increase substantially; in the others it remained stable. Serum ALP level was 69 ± 17 U/L before surgery. It remained stable during the entire preservation period and averaged 92 ± 36 U/L at 40 hours. (Fig. 7) Total bilirubin was 0.2 ± 0.1 mg/dL before surgery. It increased slightly during the preservation period, but the increase was not statistically significant. The bilirubin level was 0.3 ± 0.1 mg/dL at 44 hours. Mean portal vein pressure was 6.4 mmHg at the beginning of preservation. It increased gradually during preservation and reached 12.1 ± 1.8 mmHg at 40 hours (p<0.05). In half of the experiments, clot formation was found around the catheters placed in the portal vein. This clot formation caused incorrect pressure readings and increased portal vein pressure. Liver tissue wet/dry weight ratio was 3.65 ± 0.10, which was almost the same as that of normal dogs (3.64 ± 0.10).

Pancreatic and Duodenal Function

The pancreas and duodenum exhibited minimal functional changes during the preservation period. Secretions from these organs ranged from 1.5-8.9 ml/hour (total 60-500 ml). Serum amylase level was 1049 ± 404 U/L before surgery. It decreased slightly during the preservation period and was 839 ± 79 U/L at 40 hours. (Fig. 8) When clots formed around the catheter in the portal vein, the pancreas also appeared edematous. Tissue wet/dry weight ratio for the duodenum was 5.12 ± 0.50 after preservation, which was higher than that of normal dogs (4.19 ± 0.12, p<0.025). Tissue wet/dry ratio for the pancreas was 4.42 ± 0.20 after preservation, which was also higher than that of normal dogs (3.85 ± 0.19), but this difference was not statistically significant.

Renal Function

Total urine output ranged from 1600-2700 ml during the preservation period;

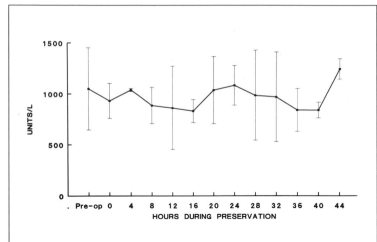

Fig. 8. Changes of serum amylase levels during the preservation period.

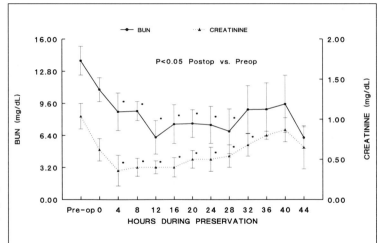

Fig. 9. Changes of blood urea nitrogen (BUN) and creatinine levels during preservation.

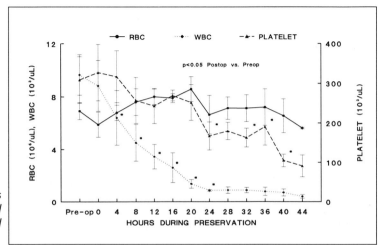

Fig. 10. Changes of blood cells during preservation. RBC: red blood cell; WBC: white blood cell; HB: hemoglobin.

hourly urine production averaged from 28-61 ml. Urine output was mainly related to the volume of fluid infusion. In the early hours, urine output was usually higher because of fluid replacement during harvesting. Kidney function was well maintained during the preservation period. Blood urea nitrogen (BUN) was 13.9 ± 1.4 mg/dL before surgery. It decreased to 8.8 ± 1.9 mg/dL at 4 hours (p<0.025) and remained at or below this level during the preservation period. It was 6.17 ± 0.08 mg/dL at 44 hours (p<0.05). Serum creatinine level was 1.0 ± 0.2 mg/dL before surgery. It decreased to 0.4 ± 0.2 mg/dL at 4 hours (p<0.01) and remained near this level during the preservation period. Serum creatinine level was 0.6 ± 0.3 mg/dL at 44 hours. (Fig. 9) The kidneys usually maintained good shape with slight edematous changes after more than 24 hours of preservation. No premature renal failure occurred in this group. Renal tissue wet/dry wright ratio was 5.89 ± 0.26 after preservation, which was higher than that of normal dogs (4.74 ± 0.16, p<0.0025).

Hematology Study

RBC concentrations were kept stable during preservation by blood or plasma transfusions. No heparin was used, and bleeding rarely occurred even though the dissection was extensive. Mean RBC concentration was 6.92 ± 0.64 (10^6/μL) before harvesting. It decreased immediately after surgery but increased during the preservation period. Mean RBC concentration was 8.58 ± 0.94 (10^6/μL) at 20 hours. Blood hematocrit levels exhibited changes similar to those in RBC concentrations. The RBC counts and hematocrit levels tended to increase because of the exudation of lymph. Plasma infusion was necessary in all experiments to keep hematocrit at normal levels. A significant reduction in WBC counts occurred during the preservation period in this study. The WBC count was 9.66 ± 1.52 (10^3/μL) before harvesting. It decreased to 0.86 ± 0.06 (10^3/μL) at 24 hours (p<0.0005) and decreased further to 0.40 ± 0.14 (10^3/μL) at 44 hours (p<0.0001). The blood platelet level was 309 ± 58 (10^3/μL) before harvesting. It decreased gradually during the preservation period; at 40 hours the level was 104.8 ± 15.9 (10^3/μL). (p<0.01, Fig. 10)

Blood Chemistry

Serum potassium, calcium, and glucose were replaced by intravenous transfusion as needed to maintain normal levels. The serum potassium level was 2.9 ± 0.5 mMol/L before surgery. It was maintained at 1.7 ± 0.3 to 2.4 ± 0.9 mMol/L during the preservation period. In our pilot study using DADLE, the heart was also very sensitive to higher concentrations of potassium. On the other hand, a relatively lower serum potassium level did not cause much difficulty. In this study, we intentionally kept serum potassium at a relatively lower level to reduce the possibility of ventricular fibrillation. Serum sodium was 151 ± 6 mMol/L before surgery. It decreased slowly during the preservation period and was 116 ± 2 mMol/L at 44 hours. The serum chloride level also decreased slightly during the preservation period. The serum total calcium level was 9.8 ± 0.9 mg/dL before surgery. It remained at a slightly lower level during the preservation period and was 8.8 ± 2.5 mg/dL at 40 hours. (Fig. 11) Blood glucose levels were usually higher than normal during the preservation period because of glucose infusions to the organ block.

Pathology Study

Some of the lung tissue samples were studied by electron microscope. Good tissue preservation for up to 40 hours was revealed. Moderate interstitial widening caused by edema was observed at 40 hours. (Fig. 12) Good tissue preservation of the heart, liver, pancreas, duodenum and kidney was also observed at 36-44 hours.

Metabolism of DADLE

In an attempt to track the metabolism of DADLE, we infused 7.5 mg of ^{125}I-labeled DADLE into the inferior vena cava and imaged the multiorgan system using a Siemens Gamma Camera Scanner. Within minutes the heart and liver had the highest concentrations of ^{125}I-labeled DADLE. Two hours later, most of the ^{125}I-labeled DADLE was secreted via the bile and, to a much lesser degree, via the urine. Only a small trace of ^{125}I-labeled DADLE could be seen in the heart and liver. The lungs did not accumulate any

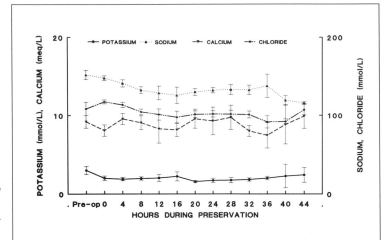

Fig. 11. Changes of serum potassium, sodium, chloride, and calcium during preservation.

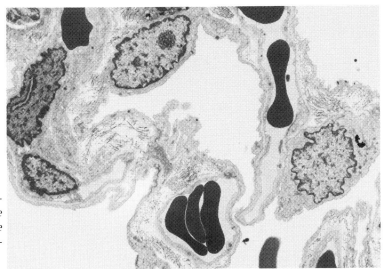

Fig. 12 A&B. Electron microscope study of lung tissue samples taken at 20 (middle photo) and 40 hours of preservation (bottom photo).

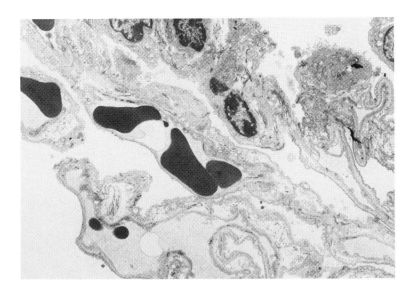

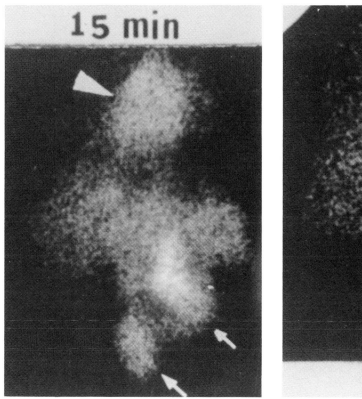

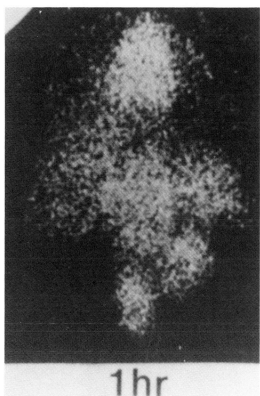

Fig. 13. [124]I-labeled DADLE distribution 15 minutes and 60 minutes after intravenous injection.

[125]I-labeled DADLE during the procedure. (Fig. 13)

THE EFFECT OF DADLE ON PLATELET AGGREGATION

The effect of DADLE on platelet aggregation was studied in one dog during the preservation period. Platelets behaved normally prior to DADLE infusion, with a dose-response relationship between the amount of adenosine diphosphate (ADP) added and the extent of aggregation. However, after DADLE infusion, even though the platelets aggregated normally in response to ADP, the platelets disaggregated shortly after ADP-stimulated aggregation, despite the use of high doses of ADP, as shown in Figure 14. A similar experiment was performed in another dog study. The particles were induced by the trauma of a laparotomy. The blood in the inferior vena cava was imaged by high resolution ultrasound before and at 20 and 60 minutes after drug administration. DADLE was infused intravenously at a concentration of

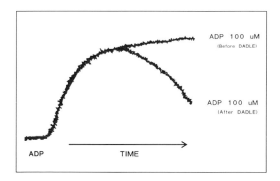

Fig. 14. The effect of DADLE on platelet aggregation.

1 mg/kg. The particles were counted and sized, and their brightness was determined. The product of these numbers is termed the "aggregate score." The aggregate score was 66,764 before DADLE and fell to 9,847 20 minutes after DADLE infusion, which appeared to represent the peak effect. The aggregate score was 30,968 at 60 minutes after DADLE infusion.

DISCUSSION

In the previous chapter, hibernation induction trigger (HIT) was found to effectively increase tissue survival time in the multiorgan preservation block. In previous studies it was also found that infusing HIT into primates induced hypothermia, aphagia, bradycardia, reduction of creatinine clearance, and lower urine flow.[1,3] Studies of blood and circulatory changes in hibernators have also found that, in hibernation, erythrocytes showed increased resistance to hemolysis.[4] Liver glycogen phosphorylase activity was strongly depressed during both short- and long-term hibernation.[5] The opiate antagonists naloxone or naltrexone either reversed or retarded these alterations.[2,6] The possible involvement of opioid receptors in hibernation has also been implicated in several other studies.[7-9] Bruce et al[10] demonstrated that continuous subcutaneous administration of naloxone, an antagonist for μ, k and δ opioid receptors, diminished the frequency and length of hibernation bouts induced by injecting plasma from winter-hibernating animals into ground squirrels (*Citellus tridedemlineatus*). This indicates that natural winter-hibernation may be induced by a mechanism involving an endogenous opioid that acts through binding to receptor sites. However, naloxone did not reverse the depression of contractility of guinea pig ileum caused by HIT from bears. This indicates that HIT itself is not an endogenous opioid.

The study by Oeltgen et al[2,11] found that infusing morphine, a μ opioid agonist, into summer-active ground squirrels caused an insignificant bout of hibernation of extremely short duration, if any.[1] Similar results were obtained with a peptidic μ opioid, morphiceptin, a naturally occurring k peptide of

brain origin dynorphin A, and a highly selective synthetic k opioid U69593.[1,9] On the contrary, HIT effectively induced animals into hibernation. However, when HIT was injected into animals that had received morphine through osmotic pumps, the hibernation-inducing effect of HIT was almost completely attenuated. The δ opioid, DADLE, exhibited completely different effects from the previously mentioned opioids in summer-active ground squirrels. Animals implanted with pumps containing DADLE began hibernating five days after implantation. DADLE did not antagonize hibernation induced by HIT. The percent frequency of hibernation induced by DADLE alone was in fact no less than that induced by a 10-mg intrasaphenous injection of HIT. The results strongly suggested that δ opioid receptor and its ligand are intimately involved in the induction of animal hibernation. Thus, the hibernation-induction property of δ opioid was relatively selective in that μ and k opioids such as morphine, morphiceptin, and dynorphin A all failed to exert the same effect.[2]

Previous studies have provided evidence that δ opioid receptors may be responsible for naturally occurring animal hibernation: 1) δ opioid receptor ligands such as DADLE have been shown to induce many physiological changes which may favor hibernation; and 2) the naturally occurring δ opioid receptor ligand methionine-enkephalin, although possessing an affinity for the μ receptor, was found to be ten times higher in concentration in the brains of deeply hibernating ground squirrels than in the brains of squirrels experiencing short-term arousals during the whole period of winter hibernation.[1]

The results of the present study demonstrated that DADLE extended tissue survival time in a very similar way as did HIT. However, the mechanism of the extension is not yet clear because of relatively insufficient studies on these very complex opioid peptides and their receptors and because of varied effects under different physiologic conditions.

The elucidation of the structure of morphine at the turn of the 19th century was followed by intensive pharmaceutical, chemical, biological and medical research into natural and synthetic opiate compounds. Despite nearly 200 years of research into the chemistry and biological actions of opiate, this field remains one of the most extensively studied areas today.[12] Since the discovery of the enkephalins in 1975, an increasing number of larger opioid peptides have been isolated. All these opioid peptides belong to one of three peptide families, each deriving from a distinct precursor molecule: proopiomelanorcortin (POMC), the common precursor for δ-endorphin, ACTH, and additional MSH-containing peptides; proenkephalin A, the common precursor for met- and leu-enkephalin and several larger enkephalin-containing peptides, e.g., peptide E, peptide F; and proenkephalin B (prodynorphin), another precursor for leu-enkephalin and for larger opioid peptides, e.g., the dynorphins, neo-endorphins and leu-morphin. The structures of these precursor molecules of several species have been determined using recombinant DNA techniques.[13] In addition to the multiplicity of opioid peptides, there is pharmacological evidence for multiple opioid receptors.[14] Studies of the binding of opioid drugs and peptides to specific sites in the brain and other organs have suggested the existence of perhaps as many as eight subtypes of opioid receptors.[15]

At least four major subtypes of the opiate receptor have been identified on the basis of their different pharmacologic profiles. In addition, biochemical and autoradiographic studies have demonstrated that these receptors are distributed differentially throughout the central nervous system and its periphery. These observations have led to the suggestion that the different opiate receptors may mediate the different pharmacologic effects of the opioids.[16] These receptors have been classified as morphine-like (μ), ketocyclazocine-like (k), N-allylnormetazocine-like (σ), and methionine-enkephalin-like (δ). However, the opioid receptors are still poorly defined because techniques are still relatively crude and because the biological functions mediated by the various opioid receptor types are not understood.[17] Recent studies have also shown that there are multiple opioid binding sites in the receptors[18]. The function of each receptor is different. The μ receptor, for which the prototypic agonist is morphine, is associated with bradycardia, miosis, respiratory deceleration, indifference and analgesia. In contrast, the σ receptor is associated with tachycardia, mydriasis, respiratory acceleration and delirium; its prototypic agonist is SKF 10047 (N-allylnormetazocine). The k receptor is associated with miosis, analgesia, sedation, and little change in pulse or respiratory rate; its prototypic agonist is ketocyclazocine.[16] The current prototypic agonist for the δ receptor is D-Ala^2-D-Leu^5-enkephalin (DADLE). However, DADLE is only three times more selective for the δ site than for the μ receptor.[16] Because opioid interactions with the circulations are highly complex, and because multiple receptors and different binding sites exist, the action of opioid agonists and antagonists may show substantial disparities. Furthermore, it appears that there is also considerable variability between species in both the specificity and selectivity of opioid receptors. For example, naloxone lowers body temperature in mice, whereas naltrexone has this effect in man. Naltrexone does not significantly alter body temperature in dogs. The changes produced by naltrexone are modest. These results suggest that endogenous ligands may play a significant role in temperature regulation in some species but a lesser role in others.[18]

The analgesic activity of opioids has been relatively confirmed in various studies. This analgesic effect may be involved in the reduction of tissue metabolism. An animal's response to noxious stimuli can be attenuated or inhibited by the injection of microgram amounts of opioids into the cerebral ventricles, into certain nuclei of the brain stem, and into the subarachnoid space of the spinal cord. These findings suggest that systemically administered opioids produce analgesia by acting at sites within the CNS. This conclusion is supported by studies demonstrating that the analgesia produced by systemically administered opioids can be antagonized by microinjection of opioid antagonists in the cerebral ventricles, the subarachnoid space of the spinal cord or brain stem nuclei.[16] However, studies have also shown that the baseline status of animal or human experiments requires careful scrutiny in formulating concepts concerning the peptide's physiologic roles. Barbiturate anesthesia completely reverses the pressor effects of leu-enkephalin on the circulation. It is clear that the same peptide could produce opposite effects under varying conditions, such as surgical manipulation, drug interaction, or route of administration.[19] It is difficult to pinpoint the exact result when peptides are used in different settings.

In this study, the heart rate was much slower than in the normal animal, and the heart continued to function during the preservation period. Blood pressure was well maintained without the help of inotropic drugs. Normal heart function was maintained throughout the preservation period as shown by stable pressures, heart rate, left ventricular dp/dt and absence of arrhythmias. There was minimal change in the color of the heart. The size of the heart was only slightly increased after 40 hours of preservation. Although the pericardium was intact in all of the experiments, no fluid was found in the pericardium at the end of the experiment. Very little change was seen in wet/dry weight ratios at the end of the experiments; these ratios were not higher than those of normal dog hearts. Isotope studies demonstrated the accumulation of DADLE in the heart early after injection, strongly indicating the direct involvement of DADLE receptors in the heart. The result was in agreement with our findings during preservation. The behavior of the heart treated by DADLE showed signs of an analgesic effect. However, this effect must have been the result of direct reactions instead of whole body regulation.

The heart treated with DADLE was also very sensitive to high levels of serum potassium. This finding is very similar to those of the HIT study. The mechanism of this high sensitivity is not yet clear. One possible explanation is related to the regulation of calcium in the heart. The fundamental contraction process, whereby cross-bridge formation between the myosin heads and binding sites on the actin filaments is activated by Ca^{++}, is the same for both skeletal and cardiac muscles. Removal of the intracellular Ca^{++} in contact with the myofibrils to a level below 10^{-7} M

results in loss of Ca^{++} from the troponin-binding sites. The result is inhibition of actomyosin-ATPase activity, breaking of the cross-bridge attachments, and relaxation of the muscle.[20] Studies have shown that several synthetic opiates can dose-dependently attenuate Ca^{++}-induced contractions of blood vessels.[21,22] It is possible that DADLE could interfere with the inflow of calcium during myocardial contraction, resulting in a relaxation of myocardium. In this way, any small increase in potassium level would augment the inhibition of myocardial contraction. In our pilot studies using DADLE, when the heart was arrested by a relatively higher level of potassium, the entire heart was totally relaxed, and resuscitation was usually unsuccessful. Our experience taught us to avoid potassium infusion. If potassium is required, it should be infused intravenously in a separate solution containing a low concentration (0.05% or less) of potassium.[23] However, the specific relationship between DADLE and myocardial performance still needs further study.

The analgesic activity of opioids was initially attributed to activation of the μ receptor. This hypothesis was based in part on the differential distribution of the opiate receptor subtypes in the brain and on the finding that regions involved in processing nociceptive information were enriched in μ sites.[16] The analgesic activity of δ agonists, particularly after intracerebraventricular or intrathecal administration, has been demonstrated in several studies, as has the existence of δ receptors in regions of the CNS involved in the processing of nociceptive information. Thus, it appears that the analgesic activity of opioids cannot be attributed to the activation of one particular subtype of the opiate receptor.[16] As a general rule, the central distribution of opiate peptide-containing cell bodies and axons follows directly the distribution of opiate receptors. In the periphery, enkephalin is localized to specific spinal regions such as the intermediolateral horn, the origin of the cell bodies of preganglionic, parasympathetic neurons. Enkephalin is also present in sympathetic ganglia; sympathetic neurons; noradrenergic vesicles; small, intensely fluorescent cells; and glomus cells of the carotid body. It is at these peripheral sites, as well as in the brain stem, that enkephalin may influence autonomic control of cardiopulmonary function.[19] Opioids stereospecifically produce hypotension and bradycardia by decreasing sympathetic tone while increasing vagal tone at autonomic nuclei of the brain stem.[19] In the study by Holaday, following third-ventricular injection in anesthetized rats, DADLE produced severe hypotension and a decrease in pulse pressure that could have been caused by δ opioid receptor actions upon decreasing sympathetic outflow.[24] The special feature in this study is that no part of the central nervous system is involved in the regulation of hemodynamics or metabolism. The only effect DADLE could produce was through peripheral action. Little work has been done in this area. In fact, the location of opiate receptors in the periphery is not well resolved. It has been demonstrated that the vagus nerve contains opiate receptors that are transported along axons from cell bodies in the nodose ganglia to the brain and the periphery. Pharmacologic evidence suggests that pulmonary "J" receptors in the lung may contain opiate binding sites. Vascular beds may also contain opiate receptors; however, specific vascular binding of opiates has not been reported. Although a small amount of opiate binding has been demonstrated in the heart, studies with whole heart homogenates have revealed that these binding sites are not stereospecific.[25]

As stated in the previous chapter, when dogs are used for organ preservation studies, severe liver congestion, which usually occurs early in the experiment and worsens during preservation, is a distinct problem. Liver congestion reduces venous inflow and effective circulating volume. The whole system deteriorates when severe liver congestion is present, despite good function of other organs. As mentioned in the previous chapter, the mechanism of this congestion is not yet totally clear. Studies have shown that the liver and portal vein bed can store large amounts of blood (as much as 30% of the total mass of blood in rabbits) and that the rate at which such stored blood is poured into the inferior vena cava is a mathematical determinant of

the amount of blood delivered to the heart. This means that the control of the outflow of blood from the livers of healthy human beings is a major factor in the control of cardiac output.[26-28] The ability of the portal vein to store blood was immediately abolished in all cases in which the innervation of the liver was destroyed.[28] The control of this reservoir mechanism was related to the existence of sphincters in the hepatic vein. In the study of Moreno et al,[29] it was shown that the sphincter located where the hepatic vein enters the vena cava contracted tightly upon stimulation. Local administration of epinephrine prior to stimulation completely prevented contraction of the hepatic vein sphincters. However, the same dose of epinephrine given after the sphincter mechanisms were set in operation failed to release the already contracted sphincters.[29] The effects of DADLE on releasing this contraction was dramatic. In all the experiments, liver congestion was minimal or absent during the operation. Even when liver congestion occurred during the preservation period, intravenous injection of DADLE eliminated congestion and restored normal function quickly.

Experimental data related to the direct effect of opioid are scarce. Direct in vivo microcirculation studies and a few in vitro studies have indicated that, depending upon blood vessel and vascular region, acute administration of opioid peptides can exert excitatory, depressant, or no effects on vascular smooth muscle.[30-32] In situ microcirculatory studies on rat mesentery indicated that, regardless of the route of administration, a variety of peptides dose-dependently dilate both terminal arterioles and precapillary sphincters. The dilation can be as much as 100% over control lumen sizes.[22,33] Using a dog hindlimb model, Caffrey et al also found that enkephalin produced hypotensive responses in anesthetized dogs.[34] We can speculate that there are opioid receptors in the hepatic vein system. The administration of DADLE dilated the hepatic vein via the receptors as shown in isotope studies. However, the exact type and location of these receptors are still not known.

Laboratory tests showed that the levels of

liver-related enzymes, mainly AST and ALT, increased immediately after the operation, then decreased during the preservation period. They increased again after 40 hours of preservation. The pattern of the increase was very similar to that seen in the HIT study. However, in only one experiment did AST and ALT increase dramatically. These enzymes were relatively low up to the end of the study in all other experiments. We believe the first increase was caused by surgical manipulation, including the damage to skeletal muscles and other organs. The second increase was caused by overall deterioration of the liver.

The quality of lung preservation was also very impressive in the study. Lung functions were well maintained up to 44 hours. No pulmonary edema was noted before 40 hours. However, lung color changes usually occurred earlier than functional changes. The earliest one occurred at 24 hours; the latest color change began at 40 hours. These changes included discoloration of the surface, red spots and local atelectasis. The change of color was mainly related to surface exposure to air during harvesting. The damage did not disappear during preservation. Lung tissue wet/dry weight ratios exhibited very little change before 40 hours.

Using a number of techniques, investigators have shown that opioids alter respiratory rate, rhythmicity, pattern and minute volume. Morphine has been demonstrated to affect independently the frequency and tidal volume control mechanisms of the respiratory center and to depress the peripheral hypoxic drive to respiration. Opioids also decrease responsivity to CO_2. For example, morphine, pentazocine, and nalbuphine shift the CO_2 stimulus-respiratory response curve in humans to the right. Opioid peptides such as [Met]enkephalin, ß-endorphin, and DADLE also depress respiration. Studies have also indicated that the respiratory depressant and analgesic effects of opioids are mediated by different opiate receptors. The effects cannot be attributed to activation of one particular opiate receptor subtype. Both μ and δ opiate receptors are involved in the respiratory depression.[16] However, these effects occur primarily through the central nervous system. Our isotope study did not indicate any binding of DADLE in the lungs, indicating the lack of δ and μ receptors in lung tissue. These preliminary results indicate that the mechanism by which DADLE extends lung preservation time in the multiorgan system is not through a direct reaction between DADLE and the lungs.

No premature renal failure occurred in this group. Laboratory tests for BUN and creatinine indicated good renal function during the preservation period. Good renal function is very important in long-term organ preservation because removing excessive water and metabolic wastes is vital for tissue protection. In this study, no unusual tissue edema occurred during the preservation period. This was clearly related to the kidney's removal of extra water in the circulation. Two to three liters of urine was excreted by the kidneys. If there were no kidney in the system, tissue edema would occur very soon after harvesting. In contrast to the autoperfusion preparation in which only the heart and lungs were used, good renal function kept the system in relatively normal condition and eliminated the need for sophisticated hemodialysis or cross-circulation.[35-37]

DADLE is a morphine-like opioid agonist-substance acting as an agonist primarily at μ, k, and δ receptors.[15] Therapeutic doses of morphine-like opioids produce peripheral vasodilation, reduced peripheral resistance and an inhibition of baroreceptor reflexes. Morphine and most opioids provoke the release of histamine, which sometimes plays a large role in hypotension. This effect is also shown in our study. When DADLE was given in anesthetized animals, systemic blood pressure could drop by as much as 50% of its original value. This vasodilation might help maintain renal function. Urine production was always high and BUN and creatinine levels always decreased during the preservation period. However, the overall effect of DADLE in our autoperfusion multiorgan preservation is more than just a result of vasodilation. The improvement of heart and lung function, the elimination of renal failure, and the extension of survival time all seem to suggest more extensive effects of DADLE. In the isotopic study, no DADLE was seen in the lungs, although the extension of lung preservation time was impressive.

As in the HIT study, white cell and platelet counts fell progressively during the course of the experiment. Serial lung sections also showed clumps of white cells in the vascular space. These two findings suggest the possibility that one reason for progressive organ dysfunction during the autoperfusion studies might be embolization of platelet and neutrophil aggregates in the heart, lungs, liver and kidney.

According to the preliminary studies, ultrasound detected circulating particles during the preservation period.[37] Using DADLE, the tissue survival time was dramatically extended. Our preliminary laboratory tests have also shown that platelets disaggregated after DADLE was injected. DADLE's effect on platelet aggregation, although not a large-scale effect, could provide a clue concerning the possible mechanism of multiple organ failure. Despite many studies, the etiology, mechanism, and treatment of multiple organ failure (MOF) or multiple system organ failure (MSOF) are still not clear. The mortality rate in patients with MOF can be as high as 90%. MOF occurs more often after major trauma (as seen in battlefield injuries) or major surgery. If the aggregated platelet and/or leukocyte is related to the development of MOF, and if DADLE can reverse this aggregation, it would be possible to use DADLE for the treatment of MOF and save many seemingly severely damaged organs and body parts by blocking or reversing the formation of these aggregates throughout the circulatory system. Because the significance of platelet aggregation in relation to tissue survival is still controversial, its relationship to tissue damage caused by leukocytes and free oxygen radicals is not yet clear.[38-40] This result is still under further investigation in our laboratory.

As mentioned before, all these explanations are speculative; more studies performed under different conditions are needed to clarify the effect of DADLE on organ preservation. LaGamma proposed that several variables be considered when attempting to determine the "physiologic" role of exogenously applied opiate peptides in cardiovascular regulation. These include: 1) the site of injection, e.g., intravenous, intracerebral, intranuclear, etc.; 2) the state of the subject, e.g., anesthetized, agitated, acute surgical preparation; 3) the cellular location of multiple subtypes of opiate receptors; 4) the various agonist specificities for preferential binding to opiate receptor subtypes, e.g., summation effects; 5) species specificity; and 6) distinguishing between pharmacologic effects and physiologic effects of putative neurotransmitters.[19] Better characterization of the pharmacologic profiles and receptor binding specificity for different species may help resolve some of the disparities.[18]

We can speculate from these results that the possible mechanisms by which DADLE extends tissue survival time may be related to the following: 1) its inhibition on tissue metabolism, 2) its effects on reduction or elimination of liver congestion, and 3) its reduction in platelet aggregation.

It should be noted that, in this study, all the experiments were performed under nonsterile or semisterile condition. Bacterial infection was usually induced during the operation or the preservation period. Gross infection was noticed, and all deaths were eventually caused by severe infection. It is presumed that, if sterilized procedures were employed, the survival time would be much longer.

References

1. Oeltgen PR, Nilekani SP, Nuchols PA, Spurrier WA, Su TP: Further studies on opioids and hibernation: Delta opioid receptor ligand selectively induced hibernation in summer-active ground squirrels. Life Sci 1988; 43:1565-1574.

2. Spurrier WA, Oeltgen PR, Myers RD: Hibernation "trigger" from hibernating woodchucks (*Marmota monax*) incudes physiological alterations and opiate-like responses in the primate (*Macacca mulatta*). J Therm Biol 1987; 12:139-142.

3. Oeltgen PR, Spurrier WA, Bergmann LC: Hemoglobin alterations of the 13-lined ground squirrel while in various activity states. Comp Biochem Physiol 1979; 64B:207-211.

4. Spurrier WA, Dawe AR: Several blood and

circulatory changes in the hibernation of the 13-lined ground squirrel, *Citellus tridecemlineatus.* Comp Biochem Physiol 1973; 44A:267-282.

5. Storey KB: Regulation of liver metabolism by enzyme phosphorylation during mammalian hibernation. J Biol Chem 1987; 262:1670-1673.

6. Green CJ, Fuller BJ, Ross B, Marriott S, Simpkin S: Storage of organs from ground-squirrels during and after hibernation. The 20th Annual Meeting for The Society for Cryobiology 1983; 149. (Abstract)

7. Beckman AL, Llados-Edkman S, Stanton TL, Adler MW: Physical dependence on morphine fails to develop during the hibernating state. Science 1981; 212:1527-1529.

8. Oeltgen PR, Walsh JW, Hamann SR, Randall DC, Spurrier WA, Myers RD: Hibernation "trigger": opioid-like inhibitory action on brain function of the monkey. Pharmacol Biochem Behav 1982; 17:1271-1274.

9. Oeltgen PR, Welborn JR, Nuchols PA, Spurrier WA, Bruce DS, Su TP: Opioids and hibernation. II. Effects of kappa opioid U69593 on induction of hibernation in summer-active ground squirrels by "hibernation induction trigger" (HIT). Life Sci 1987; 41:2115-2120.

10. Bruce DS, Cope GW, Elam TR, Ruit KA, Oeltgen PR, Su TP: Opioids and hibernation. I. Effects of naloxone on bear HIT's depression of guinea pig ileum contractility and on induction of summer hibernation in the ground squirrel. Life Sci 1987; 41:2107-2113.

11. Margreiter R, Prior C, Kornberger R, et al: Heterotopic heart transplantation. Transplant Proc 1987; 19:4375-4376.

12. Feuerstein G: The opioid system and central cardiovascular control: analysis of controversies. Peptides 1985; 6 (Suppl. 2):51-56.

13. Höllt V: Opioid peptide processing and receptor selectivity. Ann Rev Pharmacol Toxicol 1986; 26:59-77.

14. Martin WR, Eades CG, Thompson JA, Huppler RE, Gilbert PE: The effects of morphine- and nalorphine-like drugs in the nondependent and morphine-dependent chronic spinal dog. J Pharmacol Exp Ther 1976; 197:517-532.

15. Jaffe JH, Martin WR: Opioid analgesics and antagonists. In: Goodman and Gilman's the pharmacological basis of therapeutics. 7th ed. New York: MacMillan Publishing Co., 1985:491-531.

16. Hammond D: Biological effects of opioids. In: Lenz GR, Walters DE, Evans SM, Hopfinger AJ, Hammond DL, eds. Opiates. New York: Academic Press, 1986:29-44.

17. Lurie KG, Billingham ME, Masek MA, et al: Ultrastructural and functional studies on prolonged myocardial preservation in an experimental heart transplant model. J Thorac Cardiovasc Surg 1982; 84:122-129.

18. Martin WR: Pharmacology of opioids. Pharmacol Rev 1984; 35:283-323.

19. LaGamma EF: Endogenous opiates and cardiopulmonary function. Adv Pediatr 1984; 31:1-41.

20. Little RC: Physiology of the heart and circulation. Chicago: Year Book Med.Pub., Inc., 1977.59-72.

21. Altura BM, Altura BT, Carella A, Turlapaty PDMV, Weinberg J: Vascular smooth muscle and general anesthetics. Fed Proc 1980; 39:1584-1591.

22. Altura BT, Gebrewold A, Altura BM: Comparative actions of narcotics on large and microscopic blood vessels. Fed Proc 1978; 37:471. (Abstract)

23. Chien S, Oeltgen PR, Diana JN, Shi X, Nilekani SP, Salley R: Two-day preservation of major organs with autoperfusion and hibernation induction trigger. J Thorac Cardiovasc Surg 1991; 102:224-234.

24. Holaday JW: Cardiorespiratory effects of μ and δ opiate agonists following third or fourth ventricular injections. Peptides 1982; 3:1023-1029.

25. Holaday JW: Cardiovascular effects of endogenous opiate systems. Ann Rev Pharmacol Toxicol 1983; 23:541-594.

26. Krogh A: The regulation of the supply of blood to the right heart. Skand Arch Physiol 1912; 27:227-248.

27. Krogh A: On the influence of the venous supply upon the output of the heart. Skand Arch Physiol 1912; 27:126-140.

28. Knisely MH, Harding F, Debacker H: Hepatic sphincters. Science 1957; 125:1023-1026.

29. Moreno AH, Rousselot LM, Burchell AR,

Bono RF, Burke JH: Studies on the outflow tracts of the liver: II. On the outflow tracts of the canine liver with particular reference to its regulation by the hepatic vein sphincter mechanisms. Ann Surg 1962; 155:427-433.

30. Altura BT, Altura BM: Morphine actions on isolated vascular smooth muscles. Physiologist 1976; 19:109. (Abstract)

31. Flaim SF, Vismara LA, Zelis R: The effects of morphine on isolated cutaneous canine vascular smooth muscle. Res Commun Chem Pathol Pharmacol 1977; 16:191-194.

32. Lee CH, Berkowitz BA: Stereoselective and calcium dependent contractile effects of narcotic antagonist analgesics in the vascular smooth muscle of the rat. J Pharmacol Exp Ther 1976; 198:347-356.

33. Jirsch DW, Fisk RL, Couves CM: Ex vivo evaluation of stored lungs. Ann Thorac Surg 1970; 10:163-168.

34. Caffrey JL, Gu H, Barron BA, Gaugl JF: Enkephalin lowers vascular resistance in dog hindlimb via a peripheral nonlimb site. Am J Physiol 1991; 260:H386-H392.

35. Stewart RW, Morimoto T, Golding LR, Harasaki H, Olsen E, Nose Y: Canine heart-lung autoperfusion. Trans Am Soc Artif Int Organs 1985; 31:206-210.

36. Yamada T, Bosher LH, Richardson GM: Observations on the autoperfusion heart-lung preparation. Trans Am Soc Artif Int Organs 1965; 11:192-196.

37. Mahony C, Spain MG: Association of platelet and neutrophil aggregates with spontaneous contrast by echocardiography in dogs. Circulation 1986; 74 (Suppl. II):144-144. (Abstract)

38. Clark IA: Tissue damage caused by free oxygen radicals. Pathology 1986; 18:181-186.

39. Ward PA, Till GO, Kunkel R, Beauchamp C: Evidence for role of hydroxyl radical in complement and neutrophil-dependent tissue injury. J Clin Invest 1983; 72:789-801.

40. Bando K, Teramoto S, Tago M, et al: Oxygenated perfluorocarbon, recombinant human superoxide dismutase, and catalase ameliorate free radical induced myocardial injury during heart preservation and transplantation. J Thorac Cardiovasc Surg 1988; 96:930-938.

CHAPTER 6

THE EFFECT OF HIBERNATION INDUCTION TRIGGER ON HEART SURVIVAL TIME DURING HYPOTHERMIC STORAGE

In Chapter 4, we reported that using plasma from hibernating woodchucks in an autoperfusion multiorgan preparation could extend tissue survival time substantially. Several possible mechanisms were suggested for the beneficial effect of HIT on tissue survival. Among all the possible mechanisms, only the inhibition of metabolism can be seen during hypothermic storage. This study was designed to evaluate the effect of HIT on hypothermic heart storage.

MATERIAL AND METHODS

ANIMALS USED

Twenty New Zealand white rabbits of either sex weighing 4-5 kg were used. In the study group (N=10), 2 ml of HIT-containing plasma was given intravenously one day before the operation. The plasma was obtained from a deeply hibernating black bear (*Ursus americanus*) weighing 435 lbs. Another 2 ml of plasma was given 1 hour before the operation. In the control group (N=10), the same amount of normal saline but no HIT-containing bear plasma was used.

SURGICAL TECHNIQUE

Anesthesia was induced with sodium pentobarbital (30 mg/kg) IV. Heparin sodium (3 mg/kg) was infused intravenously before the operation. Artificial ventilation was induced via endotracheal intubation. With the animal in a supine position, the chest was opened through a median sternotomy. The heart was isolated, and the ascending aorta, the aortic arch, and the proximal descending aorta were dissected free. A 2 mm catheter was placed in the ascending aorta via the right innominate artery. The catheter was connected to a cylinder containing cardioplegic solution. The left subclavian artery was divided and ligated. A #2 suture was used to encircle the descending aorta for subsequent ligation. The inferior vena cava was opened, and the descending aorta was ligated. To stop the heart beat, 50 ml of preservation solution at room temperature was given through the catheter, followed by 50 ml of 4°C preservation solution. One ml of HIT-containing plasma was diluted in the final 10 ml of preservation solution in the study group. The heart was then stored in the 4°C preservation solution for 24 hours.

Composition of Preservation Solutions

The perfusion solution used was a modification of Krebs solution. It contains NaCl(120 mMol/L), KCl (6 mMol/L), $CaCl_2$ (3 mMol/L), EDTA (0.5 mMol/L), $MgSO_4$ (1.2 mMol/L), NaH_2PO_4 (1.2 mMol/L), $NaHCO_3$ (25 mMol/L) and dextrose (20 mMol/L). The preservation solution had the following composition: NaCl (120 mMol/L), KCl (20 mMol/L), $CaCl_2$ (0.8 mMol/L), $MgCl_2$ (5.2 mMol/L), KH_2PO_4 (1.2 mMol/L), $NaHCO_3$ (25 mMol/L), dextrose (20 mMol/L), mannitol (68 mMol/L) and lidocaine (0.2 mMol/L). The osmolality was approximately 350 mOsm/L.

Perfusion Apparatus

After cold storage, the heart was connected to a perfusion apparatus and placed in a temperature-controlled, humidified chamber. The setup for the apparatus is shown in Figure 1. The heart was suspended at the end of perfusion column H. The perfusion solution, which was heated at container A and bubbled with a gas mixture, was pumped by a Masterflex roller pump (Cole-Palmer, Chicago, IL). The fluid passed through a filter (K) and then went through a temperature-stabilization chamber (B). The temperature-stabilized perfusion solution then went into the perfusion line, from which the coronary artery was perfused. The rest of the fluid went into the fluid column (H), which was also temperature-controlled, and came back to the container via the overflow tubing (L). The perfusion pressure was controlled by the height of the perfusion column (H). In our study, the pressure was adjusted to 80 mmHg. The coronary return was collected by a container (D) placed underneath the heart and returned to the fluid container for recirculation. The temperature of the system, including the fluid container, the heating chamber, the perfusion column and the humidified temperature-controlled chamber, was maintained by a heating pump and circulating water. The temperature was maintained approximately 37°C during the perfusion period.

The perfusion solution was bubbled with 95% O_2 and 5% CO_2 and maintained at 37°C. A fluid-filled balloon was placed in the left ventricle through the mitral valve, which was sutured around the balloon catheter. The balloon was in fluid contact with a Gould pressure transducer (Gould, Inc, Centerville, OH). Balloon volume was started from 0 ml and increased gradually by 0.2 ml aliquots up to 1 ml. The resultant left ventricular volume, SP, EDP, and dp/dt were recorded continuously on a Gould 8-channel strip chart recorder. The coronary perfusion pressure was maintained constant at 80 mmHg during the perfusion period. Coronary flow was obtained

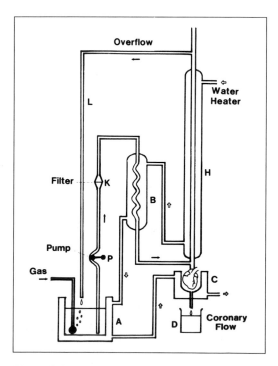

Fig. 1. Schematic drawing of the perfusion apparatus used in this study.

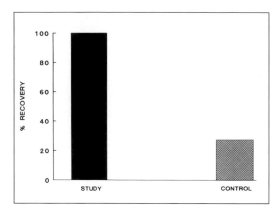

Fig. 2. Comparison of recovery of heart beat after 24 hours of hypothermic storage (p<0.001 Study Group vs. Control Group).

from the effluent of the right heart. At the end of the experiment, tissue samples were obtained from the heart for myocardial histologic and wet/dry weight ratio studies.

STATISTICAL ANALYSIS

Values obtained from the study group during the reperfusion period were compared to those from the control group at each point using ANOVA and Student-Newman-Keuls test. A value of p<0.05 was considered to indicate a significant difference.

RESULTS

After 24 hours of cold storage, all 10 hearts in the study group resumed beating following 5-10 seconds of perfusion. In the control group, only three hearts resumed beating. The other seven hearts exhibited only faint ventricular fibrillation after 1-2 hours of perfusion. (Fig. 2) In the study group, after 30 minutes of perfusion, left ventricular systolic pressure (LVSP) ranged from 33 ± 4 to 72 ± 5 mmHg when the balloon was inflated from 0.2-1 ml. Left ventricular end-diastolic pressure (LVEDP) increased to more than 25 mmHg when the balloon volume was over 1 ml. In the control group, the three beating hearts also experienced the similar blood pressure changes. After 60 minutes of perfusion, LVSP increased from 27 ± 6 to 76 ± 5 mmHg when the balloon volume was increased to 1 ml in the study group. In the control group, LVSP increased from 36 ± 13 to 81 ± 6

mmHg at 1 ml of volume. LVEDP increased from 8 ± 4 to 30 ± 6 mmHg in the study group when the balloon volume was increased to 1 ml. In the control group, LVEDP increased from 7 ± 5 to 50 ± 15 mmHg when the balloon volume reached 1 ml. (p<0.05, Fig. 3) Left ventricular generated pressure (LVSP-LVEDP) at 60 minutes of perfusion was 47 ± 6 mmHg at 1 ml in the study group, whereas in the control group this value was 24 ± 9 at the same volume. (Fig. 4) After 30 minutes of perfusion, left ventricular maximum positive dp/dt ranged from 425 ± 60 to 620 ± 111 (mmHg/second) when the balloon volume increased from 0.2 to 1 ml in the study group. In the control group, maximum positive dp/dt ranged from 433 ± 95 to 650 ± 141 mmHg/second. Left ventricular maximum positive dp/dt/p decreased from 24.5 ± 4.5 to 6.9 ± 1.6 (second^{-1}) when the balloon volume was increased from 0.2 to 1 ml in the study group. In the control group, maximum positive dp/dt/p decreased from 41.5 ± 4.7 to 8.4 ± 2.3 (second^{-1}). After 60 minutes of perfusion, maximum positive left ventricular dp/dt increased from 516 ± 60 to 920 ± 82 mmHg/second when the balloon volume was increased from 0.2 to 1 ml in the study group. In the control group, the value increased from 567 ± 192 to 683 ± 95 mmHg/second (p<0.05). Left ventricular maximum positive dp/dt/p decreased from 39.6 ± 5.6 to 22.7 ± 7.8 (second^{-1}) in the study group. In the control group, this value decreased from 24.2 ± 3.7 to 15.1 ± 2.4 (second^{-1}). (Fig. 5) After 30 minutes of perfusion, maximum left ventricular negative dp/dt increased from 277 ± 32 to 395 ± 59 mmHg/second when the balloon volume increased from 0.2 to 1 ml in the study group. In the control group, this value increased from 300 ± 24 to 500 ± 85 mmHg/second. Left ventricular maximum negative dp/dt/p changed from 17.0 ± 4.3 to 8.2 ± 1.7 second^{-1} when the balloon volume increased from 0.2 to 1 ml in the study group. In the control group, this value changed from 30.9 ± 4.5 to 14.4 ± 4.8 second^{-1}. After 60 minutes of perfusion, left ventricular maximum negative dp/dt increased from 395 ± 47 to 593 ± 69 mmHg/second when the balloon volume increased from 0.2 to 1 ml in the study group.

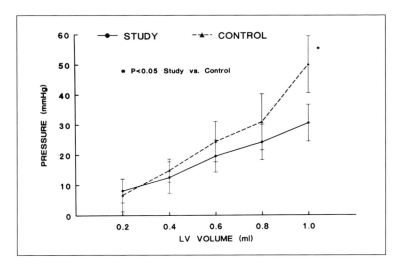

Fig. 3. Change of left ventricular end-diastolic pressure when the balloon volume in the left ventricle was increased from 0.2 ml to 1 ml.

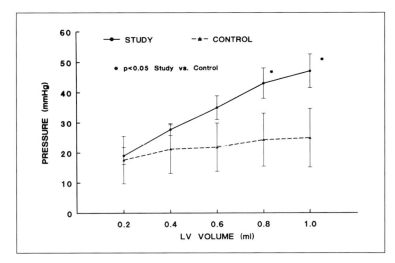

Fig. 4. Comparison of left ventricular generated pressure (systolic pressure minus end-diastolic pressure) in two groups when the balloon volume was increased from 0.2 ml to 1 ml.

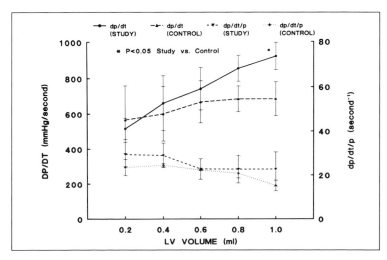

Fig. 5. Comparison of left ventricular maximum positive dp/dt and dp/dt/p in both groups when left ventricular volume was increased from 0.2 ml to 1 ml.

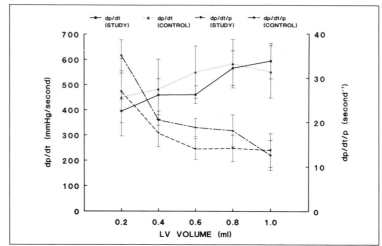

Fig. 6. Comparison of left ventricular maximum negative dp/dt and dp/dt/p when left ventricular volume was increased from 0.2 ml to 1 ml in both groups.

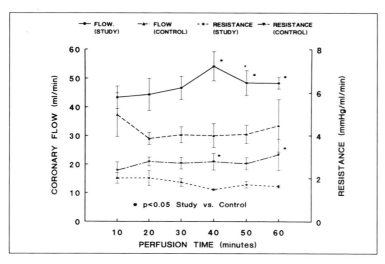

Fig. 7. Comparison of coronary flow and coronary resistance during 60-minute reperfusion in both groups.

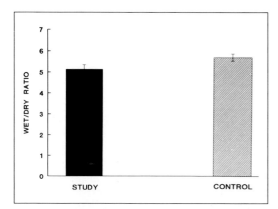

Fig. 8. Comparison of myocardial tissue wet/dry ratios after preservation in both groups (p<0.05).

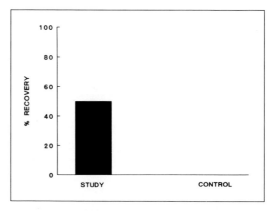

Fig. 9. Comparison of recovery of heart beat after 48 hours of hypothermic storage.

In the control group, this value increased from 450 ± 155 to 550 ± 102 mmHg/second. Left ventricular maximum negative dp/dt/p decreased from 27.0 ± 4.2 to 13.7 ± 3.8 second^{-1} when the balloon volume increased from 0.2 ml to 1 ml in the study group. In the control group, this value decreased from 35.2 ± 1.5 to 12.7 ± 3.4 (second^{-1}).(Fig. 6) Coronary flow ranged from 43 ± 4 to 54 ± 12 ml/min in the study group during the 60 minutes of reperfusion. In the control group, coronary flow ranged from 29 ± 2 to 37 ± 8 ml/min ($p<0.01$). Coronary resistance ranged from 1.48 ± 0.03 to 2.02 ± 0.25 mmHg/ml/min in the study group. In the control group, coronary resistance ranged from 2.38 ± 0.38 to 3.11 ± 0.73 mmHg/ml/min. ($p<0.05$, Fig. 7) The heart rate ranged from 111 ± 7 to 149 ± 3 bpm in the study group during the 60 minutes of reperfusion. In the control group, the heart rate ranged from 155 ± 10 to 184 ± 7 bpm ($p<0.05$). Myocardial tissue wet/dry ratio averaged 5.13 ± 0.21 for the study group and 5.68 ± 0.16 for the control group. ($p<0.05$, Fig. 8) In the study group, four hearts were stored again for another 24 hours after functional studies; two hearts resumed beating again with good pressure. In the control group, two hearts were stored for another 24 hours, but neither resumed beating. (Fig. 9)

DISCUSSION

The pioneering work of Lower and Shumway, in the early 1960s, constituted a substantial advance in the field of heart transplantation. The introduction of cyclosporine represents a further step forward. A major remaining challenge, however, is reliable preservation the graft in the interval between procurement and implantation.[1] The scarcity of donor organs is a limiting factor in heart transplantation. It has been agreed that if the problem associated with the random appearance of donors and the amount of time required to perform the transplant are to be alleviated, at least short-term preservation is necessary.[2] Multiple forms of heart preservation have been used experimentally for transplantation in the past 20 years. The first long-distance donor heart transport was performed by Thomas et al in 1978.[3] They reported that six human donor hearts were transported 203-1400 kilometers with hemodynamically successful short-term outcome in the recipients, all of whom were critically ill from end-stage cardiac failure. Extending the period of hypothermic preservation could expand the available donor pool and provide a wider safety margin for long-distance organ procurement. Four hours is currently the accepted time limit for preservation in human cardiac transplantation; longer periods of ischemia are associated with higher perioperative morbidity and mortality.[4,5]

Because of its high workload and intrinsic metabolism, the heart is very susceptible to anoxia. The maximum length of time a heart may endure ischemia and functional recovery has been studied. Studies have shown that the sudden onset of ischemia in myocardium is followed within a few seconds by a series of striking functional changes: the area becomes cyanotic and cooler; hydrogen accumulates; electrocardiographic changes appear; and within 30 to 60 seconds, contraction ceases in the affected myocardium. These changes within the ischemic focus are directly related to the development of local anoxia, which causes the affected cells to shift from an aerobic to an anaerobic form of metabolism, resulting in a substantial decrease in energy production. Although injured and nonfunctional, these severely ischemic, markedly anoxic cells are still viable and survive for a period of time. Early restoration of the coronary blood flow to an ischemic focus is followed by almost instantaneous restoration of aerobic metabolism and contractile function. However, if the period of ischemia is more prolonged, restoration of the blood supply is not followed by restoration of function, since the affected cells are either dying or dead.[6] Using an optical myograph, Tennant and Wiggers[7] documented progressive enfeeblement of contraction to the extent that within approximately one minute the area stretches during isometric contraction remains stretched during systolic ejection, and shortens quickly during isometric relaxation. Cullum et al[8] induced coronary ischemia in dogs by cross-clamping the ascending aorta.

They found that heart function was disturbed after a warm ischemic time of 30 minutes, requiring a further 30 minutes of bypass support before recovery. After 60 minutes of ischemia, satisfactory function could not be obtained after 1 hour of bypass support. The authors concluded that the safe limit of arrest with bypass support, but without drug support, lies somewhere between 30 and 60 minutes. Mitochondrial function studies performed by O'Connor et al[9] also indicated that the safe period of anoxic normothermic arrest was 30-45 minutes, and that anoxic cardiac arrest in moderate hypothermia occurred at 90-105 minutes. The morphologic changes taking place during ischemia and leading to the death of myocardial cells include relaxation of the myofibrils, progressive loss of glycogen, clumping and margination of the nuclear chromatin, and specific alterations in the mitochondria comprising an increase in matrix space, disruption of cristae, the appearance of large intramitochondrial granules, swelling and eventual rupture. The accompanying metabolic changes include insufficient production of adenosine triphosphate, loss of enzyme cofactors, accumulation of lactic acid, marked edema and electrolyte changes. These changes begin after 20 minutes of ischemia in the canine myocardium and are complete by 60 minutes when most of the cells are dead.[2,6,10]

The simplest way to control the metabolism and energy requirements is hypothermia. Hypothermia decreases the rate at which intracellular enzymes degrade the essential cellular components necessary for organ viability. Hypothermia does not stop metabolism; it simply slows reaction rates and cell death, until ultimately the organ ceases to function and loses viability.[11]

The duration of preservation achieved by reducing the metabolic rate depends on the degree of suppression. Simple hypothermia and the use of chemical metabolic inhibitors can reduce the progression of ischemic injury but cannot eliminate it. The supplementary use of pharmacologic agents will further suppress or protect the metabolism. It has also been suggested that agents that protect the integrity of cell membranes may delay ischemic damage.[2,12,13]

We have previously shown that using plasma from winter-hibernating woodchucks could extend tissue survival time in the autoperfusion multiorgan preparation.[14] We suggested the possibility that one of the mechanisms by which HIT extended tissue survival time was related to its ability to reduce metabolism.

Hibernation is a physiologic state in an endotherm characterized by depressed body temperature, respiration, cardiovascular function, and general metabolism. It is also a regulated state: hibernators avoid freezing and arouse spontaneously to euthermia and control levels of metabolism and system function.[15] Hibernation induction trigger (HIT) obtained from winter-hibernating woodchucks, ground squirrels, brown cave bats and black bears can induce hibernation in summer-active hibernators placed in a cold room. The "trigger" is not found in the blood of summer-active hibernators. Infusing a hibernation induction trigger into a non-hibernating primate induces profound behavioral and physiological depression without significant weight loss, an anesthetized state and decreased renal function. HIT has been shown to cause a significant change in renal function and creatinine clearance. In a related study by Swan and Schatte,[16] subcortical brain extracts were obtained from both winter-hibernating and summer-active ground squirrels (*Citellus tridecemlineatus*). These protein-containing extracts were injected into rats. In the rats injected with winter-hibernator brain extracts, oxygen consumption decreased to 65% of control values at 30 minutes. The observed difference between the two groups was significant up to 75 minutes. The body temperature response of the two groups was equally distinctive. After injection of brain extract from nonhibernating animals, the rats showed a mean decline of 1.5°C in three hours. In contrast, hibernating extract induced an average decrease of 5.25°C in body temperature. They concluded that hibernation of *Citellus tridecemlineatus* might be associated with the elaboration in subcortical brain tissue of an extractable agent (or agents) that depressed metabolism. The active extract could be cryogenically stored. When the agent was injected intravenously into rats, a decrease in oxygen consumption occurred, followed by a decrease in body temperature lasting from 75 minutes to 30 hours. They believed that the extract directly suppresses both metabolic rate and the subsequent thermoregulatory response.[16] It is quite possible that this brain metabolic inhibitory substance derived only from deeply hibernating ground squirrels, referred to as antabolone, might be similar or identical to the plasma-borne HIT molecule. This substance most likely has its origin from opioid-like precursor molecules of brain origin. However, this hypothesis remains to be verified by experimentation.

The results of this study show that heart function deteriorates after 24 hours of cold storage using the solution specified in this study. The results of this study are in agreement with previous reports using similar solutions. According to Belzer,[11] to be effective in hypothermic storage, the flush solution must have a composition that minimizes hypothermic-induced cell swelling, prevents intracellular acidosis, prevents the expansion of the interstitial space during the flush-out period, prevents injury from oxygen free radicals, and provides substrates for regenerating high-energy phosphate compounds during reperfusion. The solution used in this study was a relatively simple one. It does not provide all the requirements for an ideal hypothermic storage. Using continuous mechanical perfusion and a similar solution, Burt et al reported remarkable functional deterioration of hearts perfused for 24 hours.[17] In this study, when HIT-containing bear plasma was used before the operation and during preservation in the study group, heart function was better preserved than in those preservations in which HIT was not used. Hearts from the group that received HIT resumed beating after 24 hours of preservation with a very short period of perfusion. In the study group, 4 hearts were stored for another 24 hours after functional studies; half of them resumed beating after reperfusion. This was in contrast to the control group, in which none of the hearts resumed beating after a second storage period. In the studies reported by Bruce et

al,[15,18,19] blood from winter-torpid black bears (*Ursus americanus*) induced summer hibernation in 13-lined ground squirrels. Blood from polar bears (*Ursus maritimus*) was equally effective in this regard. Summer hibernation in the test species was successfully induced after intrasaphenous injection of serum from female winter-hibernating polar bears. The squirrels which received continuous low-dosage saline infusion hibernated significantly more than the squirrels with slow naloxone infusions. The results indicated the opioid nature of HIT, which may either be a precursor to or a releaser of endogenous opiate.

The ideal conditions during hypothermic storage should reduce cellular metabolism to a minimum while maintaining organelle and cellular integrity. However, significant derangements in cellular metabolism will still occur as a result of ischemia. The preservation solution should enhance the benefits of hypothermic storage by reducing ionic concentration gradients, reducing cellular and interstitial swelling, and maintaining acid-base neutrality.[20] Ultrastructural analysis demonstrated that, in hearts preserved for longer than four hours, chronic fibrosis occurred; this was considered to be the ultimate limiting factor for prolonged hypothermic cardiac preservation in man.[21] Recent development of the University of Wisconsin solution has been shown to provide longer periods of preservation time in experimental settings.[22-25] We believe that preservation time will be further extended if more effective preservation solutions are developed. In this study, we did not use very sophisticated solutions because our main purpose was to compare the results of the solutions with and without HIT.

It remains unclear how long a heart can be preserved in hypothermic storage. Studies have shown that metabolism is not completely suppressed by temperatures above 0°C, even in the presence of chemical metabolic inhibitors. Significant active transport persists even at 0°C.[26-28] If organs are kept at 0°-4°C, although metabolism is reduced, oxygen consumption is still approximately 5% of normal. It is not possible to cool the heart sufficiently to permit prolonged storage without freezing it.[27] Hypothermia itself also has adverse effects on cell physiology.[29-31] The ATPase activity is reduced under hypothermia, which in turn alters the sodium pump activity necessary to maintain normal extracellular and intracellular ion distribution.[32] The intracellular potassium concentration is decreased, and the membrane potential disappears.[33] Chloride ions consequently enter the cell. The intracellular osmotic concentration increases, water streams into the cell, and the cell swells.[34] After the organ is transplanted, this cell swelling prevents normal blood circulation in capillaries and minor blood vessels, resulting in the so-called "no reflow" phenomenon.[35] We believe that for short periods of storage, hypothermia plus chemical metabolic inhibitors would provide satisfactory results. During this time period the heart can be transported to another center for transplantation, and the patient can be better prepared so that the surgery can be performed with better chances of success. The use of hibernation induction trigger may enhance preservation time so that the safe transportation distance can be extended. The mechanism of this effect deserves further studies.

REFERENCES

1. Petsikas D, Mohamed F, Ricci M, Symes J, Guerraty A: Adenosine enhances left ventricular flow during 24-hour hypothermic perfusion of isolated cardiac allografts. J Heart Transplant 1990; 9:543-547.

2. Armitage WJ: Heart. In: Karow AMJr, Pegg DE, eds. Organ Preservation for Transplantation. 2nd ed. New York: Marcel Dekker, Inc., 1981:577-597.

3. Thomas FT, Szentpetery SS, Mammana RE, Wolfgang TC, Lower RR: Long-distance transportation of human hearts for transplantation. Ann Thorac Surg 1978; 26:344-350.

4. Jeevanandam V, Auteri JS, Sanchez JA, et al: Improved heart preservation with University of Wisconsin solution: Experimental and preliminary human experience. Circulation 1991; 84 (Suppl. III):324-328.

5. Minten J, Segel LD, Van-Belle H, Wynants J, Flameng W: Differences in high-energy phosphate catabolism between the rat and the dog in a heart preservation model. J Heart Lung Transplant 1991; 10:71-78.

6. Jennings RB, Sommers HM, Herdson PB, Kaltenbach JP: Ischemic injury of myocardium. Ann NY Acad Sci 1969; 156:61-78.

7. Tennant R, Wiggers CJ: The effect of coronary occlusion on myocardial contraction. Am J Physiol 1935; 112:351-361.

8. Cullum PA, Bailey JS, Branfoot AC, Pemberton MJ, Redding VJ, Ress JR: The warm ischemic time of the canine heart. Cardiovasc Res 1970; 4:67-72.

9. O'Connor F, Castillo-Olivares JL, Gosalvez M, Figuera D: Effect of anoxic cardiac arrest and induced ventricular fibrillation on myocardial mitochondrial respiration and oxidative phosphorylation. J Surg Res 1975; 19:325-332.

10. Jennings RB, Baum JH, Herdson PB: Fine structural changes in myocardial ischemic injury. Arch Pathol 1965; 79:135-143.

11. Belzer FO, Southard JH: Principles of solid-organ preservation by cold storage. Transplantation 1988; 45:673-676.

12. Toledo-Pereyra LH: Heart preservation. In: Toledo-Pereyra LH, ed. Basic Concepts of Organ Procurement, Perfusion and Preservation. New York: Academic Press, 1982:301-316.

13. Southard JH, van Gulik TM, Ametani MS, et al: Important components of the UW solution. Transplantation 1990; 49:251-257.

14. Chien S, Oeltgen PR, Diana JN, Shi X, Nilekani SP, Salley R: Two-day preservation of major organs with autoperfusion multiorgan preparation and hibernation induction trigger. J Thorac Cardiovasc Surg 1991; 102:224-234.

15. Bruce DS, Darling NK, Seeland KJ, Oeltgen PR, Nilekani SP, Amstrup SC: Is polar bear *(Ursus Maritimus)* a hibernator? Continued studies on opioids and hibernation. Pharmacol Biochem Behav 1990; 35:705-711.

16. Swan M, Schatte C: Antimetabolic extract from the brain of hibernating ground squirrel, *Citellus tridecemlineatus*. Science 1977; 195:84-85.

17. Burt JM, Copeland JG: Myocardial function after preservation for 24 hours. J Thorac Cardiovasc Surg 1986; 92:238-246.

18. Bruce DS, Cope GW, Elam TR, Ruit KA, Oeltgen PR, Su TP: Opioids and hibernation. I. Effects of naloxone on bear HIT's

depression of guinea pig ileum contractility and on induction of summer hibernation in the ground squirrel. Life Sci 1987; 41:2107-2113.

19. Ruit KA, Bruce DS, Chien PP, Oeltgen PR: Summer hibernation in ground squirrels *(Citellus tridecemlineatus)* induced by injection of whole or fractionated plasma from hibernating black bears *(Ursus americanus).* J Therm Biol 1987; 12:135-138.

20. Stein DG, Permut LC, Drinkwater DCJr, et al: Complete functional recovery after 24-hours heart preservation with University of Wisconsin solution and modified reperfusion. Circulation 1991; 84 (Suppl. III):316-323.

21. Takahashi A, Braimbridge MV, Hearse DJ, Chambers DJ: Long-term preservation of the mammalian myocardium. Effect of storage medium and temperature on the vulnerability to tissue injury. J Thorac Cardiovasc Surg 1991; 102:235-245.

22. Galinanes M, Murashita T, Hearse DJ: Long-tern hypothermic storage of the mammalian heart for transplantation: a comparison of three cardioplegic solutions. J Heart Lung Transplant 1992; 11:624-635.

23. Choong YS, Gavin JB: Functional recovery of hearts after cardioplegia and storage in University of Wisconsin and in St. Thomas' Hospital solutions. J Heart Lung Transplant 1991; 10:537-546.

24. Elbeery JR, Lucke JC, Speier R, Rankin JS, VanTrigt P: Analysis of myocardial function in orthotopic cardiac allografts after prolonged storage in UW solution. J Heart Lung Transplant 1991; 10:527-536.

25. Barrios A, Fell C, Hamilton WF: Effects of lung collapse on pulmonary blood volume, flow and resistance. Am J Physiol 1959; 197:187-189.

26. Karow AMJr: The organ bank concept. In: Karow AMJr, Pegg DE, eds. Organ Preservation for Transplantation. 2nd ed. New York: Marcel Dekker,Inc., 1981:3-12.

27. Barsamian EM, Win MS, Cady B, Brown H, Collins SC: Preservation of the heart in vitro. In: Brest AN, ed. Heart s=Substitutes: Mechanical and Transplant. Springfield, Ill: Charles C Thomas, 1966:263-282.

28. Collins GM, Halasz NA: Forty-eight hour ice storage of kidneys: Importance of cation content. Surgery 1976; 79:432-435.

29. Calne RY: Organ grafts. Baltimore: The Williams & Wilkins Co., 1975.31-37.

30. Collins GM: Flush preservation. In: Pegg DE, Jacobsen IA, Halasz NA, eds. Organ Preservation: Basic and Applied Aspects. Boston: MTP Press, 1982:167-177.

31. Jacobsen IA, Kemp E, Buhl MR: An adverse effect of rapid cooling in kidney preservation. Transplant 1979; 27:135-136.

32. Martin DR, Scott DF, Downes GL, Belzer FO: Primary cause of unsuccessful liver and heart preservation: cold sensitivity of the ATPase system. Ann Surg 1972; 175:111-117.

33. Walker WF, MacDonald JS, Pickard C: Hepatic vein sphincter mechanism in the dog. Br J Surg 1960; 48:218-220.

34. Whittembury G, Proverbio F: Two models of Na extrusion in cells from guinea pig kidney cortex slices. Pflugers Arch 1970; 316:1-25.

35. Grundmann R: Fundamentals of preservation methods. In: Toledo-Pereyra LH, ed. Basic Concepts of Organ Procurement, Perfusion, and Preservation for Transplantation. New York: Academic Press, 1982:93-120.

INDEX